Sexy Women Eat

Sexy Women Eat

Secrets to Eating What You Want
and Still Looking Fabulous

DIVYA GUGNANI

HARPER

NEW YORK • LONDON • TORONTO • SYDNEY

HARPER

HarperCollins books may be purchased for educational, business, or sales promotional use. For information please write: Special Markets Department, HarperCollins Publishers, 10 East 53rd Street, New York, NY 10022.

FIRST EDITION

Designed by Eric Butler

Library of Congress Cataloging-in-Publication Data

Gugnani, Divya.
  Sexy women eat / Divya Gugnani. — 1st ed.
    p.   cm.
  ISBN 978-0-06-199882-9 (pbk.)
  1. Weight loss. 2. Women—Health and hygiene. I. Title.
  RM222.2.G783   2011
  613.2'5—dc22

                                           2010022212

11 12 13 14 15   OV/RRD   10 9 8 7 6 5 4 3 2

Author's Note

This book is written as a source of information only. The information contained in this book should by no means be considered a substitute for the advice of a qualified medical professional, who should always be consulted before beginning any new diet, exercise, or other health program.

All efforts have been made to ensure the accuracy of the information contained in this book as of the date published. The author and the publisher expressly disclaim responsibility for any adverse effects arising from the use or application of the information contained herein.

Contents

Introduction **xi**

CRAZY BUT IT WORKS

Chapter 1
Spandex and Sports Bra Optional
3

Chapter 2
Ways to Say Good-bye to 150
11

Chapter 3
A Sweet Tooth for a Firm Ass
15

Chapter 4
Fat Mess vs. Hot Dress: You Decide
25

Chapter 5
**Eating Muffins Gives
You Muffin Top**
37

Chapter 6
Supersize It
49

Chapter 7
If the Apron Fits, Wear It
63

Chapter 8
True Life
71

Chapter 9
Beyond Metamucil
77

CHEAT SHEET

Chapter 10
Serving Size Sexy
83

Chapter 11
Takeout Tactics
85

Chapter 12

Ethnic Eats

91

Chapter 13

The Four O'Clock Problem

97

Chapter 14

Room Service

105

Chapter 15

The Morning After

113

YOU CAN'T MAKE THIS STUFF UP
_____

Chapter 16

Liar, Liar, Plate on Fire

121

Chapter 17

Spot Secret

133

Chapter 18

How Not to Be a Heifer This Holiday

143

Chapter 19

A Mano Is Not a Man

149

LIFE LESSONS

Chapter 20
Office Space
155

Chapter 21
My Happy Pills
159

Chapter 22
Breakup Binge
165

Chapter 23
Food Cures All
171

Chapter 24
Mr. Martini
177

Acknowledgments   183

Sources   187

Introduction

I had a bowl-shaped haircut and buck teeth. My family called me "Beaver." Just picture an eight-year old walking down the aisle of the supermarket and her dad screaming "Beaver" across the cereal boxes. No, my parents are not perverts. They are Indian immigrants who happen to have a profound sense of patriotism and didn't realize the sexual connotation. They gave me that name because I was always as busy as a beaver (some things never change!). I've been trying to outgrow it ever since, but every now and then my sister just slips and lets it out like she's on a loud-speaker. As if my childhood pet name wasn't bad enough, I wore glasses and looked like a blind person dressed me for school each day. Why else do you think I hid in the kitchen when my parents had parties? It was time well spent, as I learned how to cook at a young age. My family is obsessed with food. At breakfast we discuss lunch, at lunch we debate dinner options, and after dinner we marinate our minds to start the drill all over again in the A.M. We have two refrigerators in our house and every time you open one of them, you are sure to get hit in the knees with a piece of falling cheese or knocked out by veggies flowing out from the overstuffed shelves. When we entertain in the winter, we park our cars in the driveway and put food in the trunk because there is never enough room in either of our refrigerators. You can put any protein, fruit, or vegetable in front of me and I will find a way to slice, dice, and sauté it.

My passion for cooking and stints in two culinary programs eventually turned into a profession after a ten-year career in finance ranging from investment banking to venture capital. After coaching many companies of all sizes on building, growing, and selling their businesses, I retired as a full-time coach and became a captain. I founded and created Behind the Burner, a culinary media brand, which allowed me to blend my passion for food and fine wine with business.

At Behind the Burner we feature a network of experts in four fields: food, wine, mixology, and nutrition. We package our experts' (celebrity chefs, winemakers, mixologists, nutritionists, etc.) best tips, tricks, and techniques in the form of videos, articles, and blogs. Our videos get syndicated on broadcast TV (NBC New York Nonstop) and a large network of online media properties. I do regular weekend programming for WNBC, and we even have a podcast on iTunes for those of you who live life via gadgets. We offer discounts on the tools and ingredients the experts recommend so you can replicate restaurant quality experiences at home, in a flash, at a fraction of the cost.

So, with my new career, I officially eat and drink for a living. I jump from city to city with my team, eating and drinking all that America (and beyond!) has to offer. Does life get better than that? I think not. With the help of braces (later InvisAlign) and Lasik surgery (thank God for both), this ugly duckling turned into a swan and smiles in front of cameras on a daily basis. Some of the best designers lend me clothes, hence masking my ineptitude to dress myself. I also stuff my face with the most delicious food, sip the season's best wines, and go bottoms-up on the latest cocktail craze.

Regardless of my job or position, I've always lived life with one philosophy: pick the job you love and it won't feel like work. Get the position that you enjoy; yes, the one that you would be happy to have even if you never got paid to fulfill your duties. Come into the office each day and give it your 100 percent. Scratch that. One million percent. Whether it was walking into 85 Broad Street at Goldman Sachs as an investment banking analyst or being a line cook on Sixty-third Street at Chef's Table, I lived each day as a sponge, ready to soak up every bit of information and learn every skill possible.

For the ten years prior to Behind the Burner, I paid my dues, climbed up the venture capital ladder, and eventually reached a point in my career where I had hours to spend in the gym (while minions crunched numbers in windowless cubicles, of course). Everything changed very quickly when I launched my own business. Just as fast as my six-figure paycheck disappeared, so did my personal time. Welcome to the life of a start-up. Good-bye happy hour with friends and hello twelve- to twenty-hour days filled with technical challenges, strategy meetings, delayed filming schedules, and much more. As a media entrepreneur at an emerging company I have zero minutes and zero seconds to dedicate to my personal well-being, therefore, the world has become my gym. Sleep is a luxury I can't afford. With a few mistakes along the way and a string of not-so-suitable suitors, I've finally learned how to be fit and fabulous while enjoying every bite of my decadent lifestyle. Furthermore, if eating sweets is wrong, then I don't want to be right.

I went from roadkill to ravishing and lucky you is about to be served my culinary secrets learned Behind the Burner.

I'm a food slut, or in simpler terms, a woman who eats. For me, sexy is ravishing. It is confidence and beauty with an honest appetite and a healthy mind-set. Not someone who dates just to eat good meals and after getting wined and dined gives the purchaser of their expensive dinners a little nooky. I know a girl's gotta eat, but believe me, ladies, it's so much tastier when you've worked hard enough to be able to afford your dining adventures. Instead, I'm a new breed of food slut; someone with a disgustingly unnatural appetite; someone who scarfs down food quicker than anyone else at the table. Yet someone who has also learned that eating is a beautiful thing that can still leave you looking and feeling fabulous. So I hope you'll turn the page and dig into my little black book of tips to keep your body fit and your stomach full.

CRAZY BUT IT WORKS

Chapter 1

Spandex and Sports Bra Optional

I Don't Sweat It When I
Can't Make the Gym

At 5:00 P.M. on a Saturday night I was riding down the company elevator (yes, we worked Saturdays), and John Corzine (former CEO of Goldman Sachs) asked me, "If I built a gym, would you use it?" My response was, "Hell yeah." Sure enough, months later, Goldman Sachs had its own gym; rock-climbing wall and all. Better yet, we got workout clothes to prevent us from schlepping them back and forth to work and having people in the subway give us appalled looks. Wondering where that dirty sock smell was coming from? Not my bag! For those two years of my life, Goldman Sachs headquarters near Wall Street was my home. Early mornings, late nights, and constant travel left me little time to actually nest in my apartment. My bed was my only furniture friend and I saw it for about four to six hours a night—

if I was lucky! Most other nights I lived the high life—you know, sleeping on a managing director's couch or my winter coat on the floor of my cubicle. My puffy North Face jacket made the best mattress, I soon discovered.

On the bright side, I must say the Goldman gym was paradise. The machines were not made of gold, although they probably could have afforded that, it was just a state-of-the-art adult paradise. I ran on the treadmill while watching all of the latest sitcoms (back in the day when it wasn't *all* reality TV) that I secretly wished I was watching on my comfy couch at home. Thank God for Netflix. I took classes and even became a decent rock climber. One day, upon returning from the gym at 8:00 P.M. and ordering the maximum allowable food for my daily corporate dinner budget, I noticed a very nice pair of Via Spiga heels in the stall next to me in the bathroom. Hours later, after cranking out more numbers than any human brain should be allowed to hold, I returnd to the bathroom and saw those Via Spiga heels in the same place. Either someone with very nice shoes was murdered in that stall, or someone had taken off her shoes and fallen asleep mid-pee (I highly doubt passing out during mid-shit was possible). I assumed it was the latter. It turns out one of my fellow analysts was taking a much needed nap on the can. She had even walked up two flights of stairs to my floor so that no one from her department would recognize her shoes!

You may think you are Superwoman, but truth be told, we all need to sleep, especially if we want to maintain our ideal weight. So, ladies, get it while you can—even if you have to nap in bathroom stalls. When you get enough sleep (and I don't), you won't rely on sweets and carb-filled snacks as much to stay awake during the workday. That means fewer calories in your belly for the day. Also, hormones affect your sleep. Two hormones, ghrelin and leptin (no, they are not gremlins), work together to control your feelings of hunger and fullness. Ghrelin stimulates your appetite and is produced in your gastrointestinal tract, while leptin tells your brain when you are full and is produced in fat cells. When you don't get enough z's, your leptin levels go down, which means your tummy doesn't feel full after you eat. Not enough sleep also causes spikes in your ghrelin, which stimulates your appetite, so you reach for all of the cookies in the cookie jar. Now, back to bathrooms . . .

Months later, one of the assistants in my group was making panting noises from the handicapped stall and I realized she was doing jumping jacks. I asked her why she didn't just go to the gym. She told me doing jumping jacks in the Goldman Sachs bathroom was all the exercise she could get as a mother of a toddler who also commuted forty minutes a day to work. Just when I thought I had it rough sleeping in a cubicle, I realized life could be worse.

For the years that followed, I didn't have the luxury of a workplace gym, but I kept up the bathroom exercise (I prefer jogging in place rather than doing jumping jacks, especially when I can't get a handicapped stall) and made a point of walking to work regularly and walking home. It allowed me time to destress, relax, and be alone with my own thoughts (scary!). If you know me, you'd know that I don't sweat much. So, lucky me, I got to work without the need to spray on perfume upon walking in the door. Because I loathe mornings, A.M. workouts in the gym are not my cup of tea. Instead, I would go home, work out, and then make myself a simple and easy dinner. No thirty-minute meals in my house. More like fifteen-minute meals or five- to ten-minute ones if I was superorganized. Daily groceries were picked up on my walk home, of course.

During the day I kept dumbbells under my desk. I'd break them out in the middle of conference calls to prevent myself from being entirely bored out of my skull. I wore ankle weights under my Theory pants. The key was that no one ever knew that I was burning more calories and building muscle with each step I took. I'd hoist myself up on the kitchen counter while heating up my lunch to get my biceps and triceps toned—talk about successful multitasking! Every now and again, someone would walk by my office and see my face bopping up and down while I did body lifts with my office chair. While my co-workers wanted to check me into the nearest insane asylum, I was just trying to stay fit in any way possible while working the heinous hours that were par for the course given my career in finance. I had turned my office into my own personal gymnasium, making use of every feasible object around me in order to stay fit. This was far from mental, it was pure genius. I felt that little spurts of exercise would get my heart rate up and help me burn off all my calorie-laden meals more efficiently. During a brief stint working in Palo Alto, California, I kept sneakers in my desk drawer and walked around our company parking lot during lunch. I took the stairs every chance I got. Trust me, if you saw my egg-cracking toned ass, you would too.

Speaking of ass, I got off mine every time I had to ask a colleague a question. In the world of e-mail, I admit to being a regular abuser, communicating via screen to people two feet away from me. Technology has made us lazy, but I still value human interaction, especially when I need to discuss important business matters that can be lost over mistyped words. Every now and again someone will notice that I'm lifting my legs constantly under my desk to tone my thighs. After all, I've got my mom's genes but clearly not her body shape, since her thighs are about half the size of mine. Some of us just have to work for it.

My favorite office gadget of all time is the headset. I couldn't live without it. I was on the phone constantly, but would pace around my office like a frantic wannabe Wall Streeter (stress ball in hand, of course) and burn calories, even while on the phone. When I drove to meetings or got dropped off, I would get out far away from the entrance, just so I could get a walk in before getting stuck in a windowless conference room for hours. These little sporadic spurts of exercise would boost my energy level and help me concentrate better all day. They also helped me get good quality sleep at night, a rarity in my life, as you know by now.

Overall, I've got a new take on fitness. It's gotta be part of your everyday life, not just two hours of a kick-ass routine with a personal trainer. A lot of my exercise occurs without having to watch overly confident men trying to lift weights that are just too heavy for them. Spandex and sports bras are not mandatory for burning a few extra calories. I prefer my exercise to be simple and not too sweaty. I have a horrible habit of multitasking while I work out. At my last venture capital firm, we had yet another company gym. I frequently took conference calls while I was climbing flights of stairs on the Stairmaster. I confess I did kill a few BlackBerries by typing e-mails and dropping them on my feet while walking on the elliptical machine. A combination of strength training (and that doesn't mean carrying your over-stuffed purse around town—that's just bad for your back) and cardio is the perfect recipe for a toned body without having to feel the burn of overdone workouts.

I also try to swim a few days a week. My father threw me into a pool when I was about two years old and I've been a fish ever since. If there is a body of water in sight, I need to be in it—minus the man-made lake at Central Park. As the CEO and host of Behind the Burner, I've found that my knees and back pretty much hate me. They suffer about four hours a day of standing in pencil-thin Jimmy Choos and Louboutins. When I'm exercising, I try to spare them and stick to swimming, which is oh so much better on my joints than running and other forms of cardio. Swimming also helps me build my endurance and power through long days of filming. It builds muscle mass, strengthens and tones muscle while protecting joints from strain and stress. Additionally, swimming forces me to wear a bikini all year long, reminding me summer isn't the only time to tighten those abs.

In the winter, people get lazy. The only walking they do is to the fridge, and strength training involves carrying lunch back to their desk. Don't fall into this trap. Even though that winter sweater hides love handles quite nicely, they will be out for public display when you take that much needed winter beach vacation. I will also admit to wearing a pedometer and tracking my steps (particularly in the winter). It's a fun experiment where I get competitive with myself and try to take as many steps as possible. I log on and monitor my steps quite obsessively. Oh, and the dorky black thing clipped on my nice shoes is a constant topic of conversation and makes the day more thrilling.

One late night, pounding away on my Mac keyboard in bed, I started watching some infomercials in the background. Okay, I'll admit, I can be a sucker. I have a Ped Egg and a few hair gadgets too! But I haven't succumbed to Bumpit yet, don't worry. Besides, my hair isn't even flat. Anyhow, what I did fall victim to was an infomercial for 10-Minute Trainer and immediately ordered it—I love how I'm referring to the trainer as some troll pet about to whip my ass in shape. But come on, who doesn't want to work out for ten minutes a day and look like they spent hours in the gym? When the package arrived at work, I tore it open and got started right away by popping the CD in my work laptop. I discovered the workouts were easy and the ten minutes just flew by. I got my heart rate up pretty significantly and I felt like it was time well spent. I mixed it up between cardio, yoga, and abs.

Over the next few months, I modified the workouts and even put in my own moves—impressive, right? I have been committed to exercising ten minutes a day about four days a week, regardless of how many restaurant openings and parties I attend on a daily basis. I made a commitment to myself that ten minutes is so little to spare.

And no, I am not some spokesperson for this workout tape. The point is simple: if I can take ten minutes to watch some catfight on a reality TV show I can definitely take ten minutes out of my day to work on my own body. And so can you.

My Seven Best Kept Nutrition Secrets, Revealed!

1. *Forget family-style:* Recent studies have found that when people are served pre-plated food as opposed to empty plates with a platter of food in the middle of the table, they eat up to 35 percent less.

2. *Pop to it!* Nutritionists have found that people who ate one cup of microwaved popcorn thirty minutes before lunch

consumed 105 fewer calories at the meal (just make sure you choose plain, lightly-salted popcorn, and hold the butter!).

3. *Meaty mushrooms:* Research reports that people who ate mushroom-based entrées felt just as satisfied as when they'd eaten those same dishes made with meat. Substituting mushrooms for meat is a great way to cut fat and cholesterol.

4. *Incredible and edible:* Eggs aren't just for breakfast—they make great additions to salad and portable snacks because they pack a punch of protein and amino acids.

5. *Slimming salads:* Did you know that eating a salad before an entrée can reduce your overall calorie intake by as much as to 12 percent?

6. *Kick the cravings:* The greatest numbers of cravings occur late in the day, when our blood sugar tends to drop. So arm yourself with a handful of nuts or a piece of fruit to snack on.

7. *Wine not?* Wine has positive effects in more ways than one. Studies show that people who drank one glass of wine a day had slimmer waistlines than those who drank no alcohol. Cheers!

Chapter 2

Ways to Say Good-bye to 150

Killing Calories the Everyday Way

A hundred and fifty calories is a piece of cake to burn off, if you actually avoid that sliver of cake. I can think of about fifteen items that are worth 150 calories—two tablespoons of mayo, a glass of soda, hummus and a few crackers, a glass of chocolate milk, small bag of popcorn, one string cheese, two celery sticks with peanut butter, etc. The point is, 150-calorie snacks are consumed every day. More important is how to burn off these 150 calories without the gym membership. Just don't be a couch potato the minute you step out of the office and your body can easily transform into a lean mean fat-burning machine—and I don't mean go out and buy a George Foreman grill either.

CLEANING: Wipe down the house blinds, vacuum, and dust for thirty minutes.

DANCING: My personal favorite, of course—dancing for thirty minutes (or a few hours if you're me after a night out) is a great exercise to burn off that margarita and the Coronas you inhaled at the bar.

SHOPPING: Trust me, the mall is the new track if you ask me. Actually if you ask any Gugnani. Walking from Macy's to Nordstrom's, if on opposite sides of the mall, is actually equivalent to walking three blocks. Never take the escalator, avoid the food court, and try to visit stores that have two or three levels so you can shop till you drop (the pounds), literally! Hold that belly tight as you walk and swing those arms like the power-walking mommies in your neighborhood. It's exhilarating.

COOKING: I know this may seem counterintuitive, but cooking for other people is actually a workout. Squeeze those glutes and chop some onions, squat down a few times to check the oven or get your pots and pans, mix some batter, and lift meat trays. The oven is the best sweat yet! Cook for about two hours without taste-testing every second and you're guaranteed to burn those calories from the bagel shop earlier that day.

JUMP: Jump rope for twelve minutes in your basement or outside. You don't need to spend your bank account on treadmills and ellipticals, people. Jumping rope and doing some crunches work just as well.

WALK: Take a relaxing stroll during your lunch break. Use twenty minutes of your lunch break to have a healthy salad or sandwich and use the remaining forty to walk around the block. It's not hard to make time for fitness, even with a full-time job. Besides, moving around is a stress reliever from the hectic nine-to-five day anyway.

SHOVEL: Don't want to break a sweat? Shovel snow for about fifteen minutes and the calories will melt off—well, maybe not melt, but you get the picture.

MORE CLEANING: Washing windows and doors for about forty minutes is a great way to burn calories. I suggest playing "Burn, Baby Burn, Disco Inferno!" It's great motivation.

STAIR MASTER: If you work on the eighth floor of an office building, why not take the stairs? Stair walking for about fifteen minutes daily does the trick. If you live in an apartment building close to the groud floor, you can keep fit by constantly opting to walk up and down the stairs.

PARK FAR AWAY: Park your car far enough away so that you get a few minutes of a cardio burst. Who cares if it's drizzling? Park farther from your destination so you have to walk that extra few minutes to get there.

WASH YOUR CAR: You don't need to spend ten bucks on a car wash every month. Instead, grab a hose, some rags and some soap, and do it yourself, lazy ass. Try to carry the buckets too. Washing any vehicle for about a half hour to an hour helps.

YARD WORK: Don't be afraid to get down and dirty to drop those pounds. Raking leaves, planting, weeding, and lawn mowing for an hour or so allow you to burn the cals while being productive around the house.

BICYCLING: Riding your bike for fifteen minutes can burn 150 calories. Everyone should own a bike, hopefully one without training wheels if you're smart enough to be reading this book. Riding for an afternoon is a whole workout in itself.

SWIMMING: Pools are both indoor and outdoor, so there is no excuse not to swim. Swimming a few laps or even exercising your legs while holding on to the side is a quick calorie burner. It will also force you to look good in a bathing suit year round.

WORKOUT AT WORK: Call me crazy, but in my book, there is absolutely nothing wrong with bringing weights to work. I have two purple rubber dumbbells of ten pounds each under my desk. During downtime—if there is any—I do some lifts. After a while, toning and typing will become a daily routine.

Chapter 3

A Sweet Tooth for a Firm Ass

Store-bought Cake? I Don't Think So

I was practically born with a chocolate chip cookie in my mouth. Unlike most people with a common sweet tooth, I've got a whole set of thirty-two candy, chocolate-craving teeth . . . soon to be dentures if I keep it up. My earliest kitchen adventures were rich double chocolate brownies, fresh-baked peanut butter cookies, and ultramoist vanilla cakes oozing with vanilla frosting. I guess that would explain why Cookie Monster had my heart over Big Bird during my *Sesame Street* days. After track practice I would tune into *Sweet Dreams* and watch Gale Gand show off her baking sensibility on the Food Network. Watching her show for nearly eight years inspired me to bake for anyone who would eat my treats; the mailman, the neighbors, my friends, my teachers (how do you think I got A's?!). My mother would try to force a cupcake down her friends' throats as soon as they walked in our door. It should come as no surprise that I would always lead the pack during the Girl Scout cookie drive. Yes, I will admit, my winning strategy was to buy at least ten boxes of Tagalongs and Thin Mints for personal consumption. During the holidays, my aunt Verna would visit us from Springfield, Illinois, and the two of us would go into pie-baking frenzy. There wasn't a piece of fruit in our home that escaped landing in a pie. By the way, I only eat the filling of pies. The crust is for the birds.

Store-bought sweets in my home? Absolutely not. Okay, I will admit to an occasional box of Entenmann's cookies when I'm feeling very lazy and particularly skinny. Baking doubles as my pleasure. What's better than eating raw batter and tasting it again when it's baked? Well, maybe raw cookie dough, despite the risk of salmonella.

All this training worked out to be quite handy for me, as we all know that every woman needs to master the art of making at least one sweet treat—mainly because there will be that moment when she needs to show off her skills and blow the pants off a very special male in her life. It may be a thank-you for all the trendy restaurants he's taken you to, or a delivery to his office to let his co-workers know he's yours, part of your recessionary dating strategy when you're low on dough, or most likely a ploy to lure him to your apartment for full-on seduction. Whatever your motive, for the modern woman knowing how to bake is as essential as a great pair of f— me shoes . . . or should I say, stilettos? And truth be told, every man deserves a custom creation. If you are feeling particularly adventurous, invite him to join in on the mixing, whipping, shaping, and baking of mouthwatering goodies. It makes for great foreplay in the bedroom too. Use your imagination!

So you're not Martha Stewart. It's okay. If you can't bake it, learn how to fake it and PUH-LEASE do it the healthy way. I mean, the point is for him to take off the apron, right? Use these tips to keep your figure fabulous and your blood sugar low, while still enjoying those baked treats. It's easy as pie.

With sweets this good, get ready to deal with full-on infatuation. You can still indulge by doing things the guilt-free way with helpful, simple tips. I asked some baking experts and nutritionists to share these secrets for my black book, and here's what I discovered, fresh out of the oven!

Fat Attack

Fat isn't the all-encompassing, secret ingredient to baked goods. Butter and oil can be replaced with other moist ingredients, such as applesauce, orange juice, light cream cheese, and fat-free sour cream. Oh and get this . . . baby food may be added to your budget this holiday season, and not because you're expecting. Use little jars of puree for replacing up to half the fat in a baking recipe. I prefer to puree it myself, but if you're lazy, grab some Gerber baby food and get busy. You can puree sweet potatoes and use them for baking cakes, pound cakes, and almond bread, or even use pureed prunes for your favorite cookie recipe.

Applesauce and plain yogurt are good fat substitutes in most recipes. I've learned that for maximum texture and flavor, replace no more than half the amount of the fat listed in the recipe. If a recipe calls for ½ cup butter, you can substitute ¼ cup applesauce, saving 44 grams of fat and 400 calories.

Depending on the baked treat you are preparing, milk can be a good alternative to butter and oil. A little reduced-fat milk can add moisture to cakes, cupcakes, and muffins. People like Jerry

Seinfeld's wife get lots of credit and acclaim for baking kiddie cuisine in this manner. I promise you won't taste the actual milk in the final product. Also, try replacing butter with coconut oil and using egg whites instead of caloric egg yolks in your batter.

One of my girlfriends swears by tofu as a substitute for fattening ingredients in desserts. She uses it to replace eggs, as a substitute for cream cheese in cheesecake, and as a base for pudding. Now, let's get real. Tofu is simply bean curd, made by coagulating soymilk and turning the rest of the soft white food into blocks. Gross, right? Wrong! Tofu provides you with high iron, low fat, rich antioxidants, and a taste just as good! It is also sold everywhere and baked goods made with tofu taste delicious. Take your favorite Russian tea cakes, banana breads, and chunky chocolate cookies and try making them with tofu. It's all about experimenting. Save your budget for fatty desserts for when you dine out and enjoy these lower-calorie healthier stunt doubles at home. I'm not saying go vegan (this isn't *Skinny Bitch*), but I am saying get creative with your goods without clogging your arteries and icing your ass with layers of extra fat.

Flour Power

Replace regular white flour with healthier kinds of flour, like almond flour, quinoa flour, or protein powder. I recommend King Arthur's White Whole Wheat Flour. It is nutritionally equivalent to whole wheat flour but with a lighter color and flavor.

Sugar Subs

You do not need to follow Betty Crocker's exact sugar dosages for every cake you bake. Use less sugar (a teaspoon instead of a tablespoon). Some people substitute a no-calorie sweetener for part of the sugar required in a recipe. Personally, I'm against Splenda, Equal, and Sweet 'n Low, so I opt for natural sweeteners like agave nectar and honey where I can.

Molasses is another option: it's a thick syrup that retains many minerals and has lower sugar content. The darker the molasses, the higher the mineral content and the lower the sugar. Molasses has a strong flavor, so it's probably best to use it as just one of the sweeteners when you are baking, rather than the sole sweetener.

Maple sugar is a great natural sweetener. It is made from the sap of maple trees. When you are buying maple syrup, skip the Aunt Jemima. Instead, spring for the real Canadian kind or the stuff from Vermont. The flavor will be far more intense and satisfying aside from the fact that you won't be ingesting as many chemicals.

A little Caribbean secret: coconut sugar is a great sugar substitute when baking. It is obtained from coconut flour buds but tends to clump, so be sure to break up any pieces before adding it to your baked goods.

Finally, date sugar can be used to replace the addictive diabetes-causing powdered sugar on most goodies. Date sugar is made from coarsely ground dried dates, is minimally processed, and retains the wonderful complex flavor of dates. It can be used in the batter of baked goods or be sprinkled on top. Similarly, I also like Sugar in the Raw.

'Tis the Season

The tree isn't the only thing to trim this holiday season. Keep your body in shape without the typical New Year's resolution diet—a.k.a. let me starve myself until next November.

When baking chocolate cookies (using snowflake cookie cutters, of course), I use cocoa powder instead of unsweetened chocolate. Also, I usually don't use the full pound of chocolate chips or Hershey kisses the recipe might recommend. We all know the full package of chocolate chips isn't quite necessary, unless you want your Christmas gift to your family to be a few extra pounds!

Now it's time to channel your domestic diva and get your sugar fix at the same time. And let that special someone get his too. Just let your better half be the bigger Cookie Monster. The object of your affection will be only too pleased. This is an adult wake and bake that your significant other is not going to want to miss. The aromas will serve as an aphrodisiac. It's what I call sweet success.

Baked Apples (Hold the Pie)

MAKES 4 SERVINGS

2 apples, cored and sliced
¼ cup brown sugar
2 tablespoons whole wheat flour
¾ teaspoon ground cinnamon
¼ teaspoon ground nutmeg
1 teaspoon vanilla extract
¼ cup chopped walnuts
¼ cup 1% milk

Nutrition Facts	
Amount Per Serving	
Calories 166.9	
Total Fat 5.5g	
Saturated Fat 0.6g	
Trans Fat 0.0g	
Cholesterol 0.8mg	
Sodium 12.7mg	
Total Carbohydrates 33.9g	
Dietary Fiber 3.1g	
Sugars 19.5g	
Protein 2.3g	
Vitamin A 1.4%	Vitamin C 6.9%
Calcium 5.0%	Iron 4.2%

1. Preheat the oven to 350° degrees F. Grease a baking dish or use a nonstick one.

2. Place the apples in a large bowl. In a small bowl, mix together the sugar, flour, cinnamon, and nutmeg. Stir the spice mixture into the apples until evenly distributed. Fold in the walnuts. Spoon into the prepared dish. Pour the milk evenly over apple mixture.

3. Cover the apples with aluminum foil before baking.

4. Bake in the oven for 45 minutes, or until soft and bubbly. Allow to cool slightly before serving.

Tip: Covering the apples with foil before baking locks in the moisture.

Crumbling Pear

MAKES 2 SERVINGS

3 pears, peeled, cored, and sliced

2 teaspoons lemon juice

3 tablespoons brown sugar

3 tablespoons old-fashioned oats

2 tablespoons whole wheat flour

¼ teaspoon ground cinnamon

Dash ground nutmeg

1 tablespoon cold butter

2 tablespoons chopped almonds

Nutrition Facts	
Amount Per Serving	
Calories 388.8	Calories from Fat 166
Total Fat 11.3g	
Saturated Fat 4.2g	
Trans Fat 0.0g	
Cholesterol 15.5mg	
Sodium 10.1mg	
Total Carbohydrates 86.4g	
Dietary Fiber 9.9g	
Sugars 29.8g	
Protein 5.0g	
Vitamin A 5.4% •	Vitamin C 19.7%
Calcium 8.2% •	Iron 12.2%

1. Preheat the oven to 350° F.

2. Place the pear slices in a greased 1-quart baking dish. Sprinkle with lemon juice.

3. In a separate bowl, combine the sugar, oats, flour, cinnamon, and nutmeg. Cut in the butter until crumbly; add the nuts. Sprinkle over the pears. Bake at 350° F for 25 to 30 minutes.

Tip: If your pears are not ripe, put them in a brown paper bag at room temperature for two to three days.

Cranberry Almond Chocolate Clusters

MAKES 12 CLUSTERS

1 cup toasted almonds,
    coarsely chopped
½ cup dried cranberries,
    coarsely chopped
6 ounces dark chocolate,
    finely chopped

Nutrition Facts		
Amount Per Serving		
Calories 136		
Total Fat 8.8g		
Saturated Fat 3.7g		
Trans Fat 0.0g		
Cholesterol 4mg		
Sodium 13mg		
Total Carbohydrates 12.0g		
Dietary Fiber 1.7g		
Sugars 9.0g		
Protein 3.0g		
Vitamin A 1%	•	Vitamin C 1%
Calcium 5%	•	Iron 4%

1. In a bowl, mix the almonds and cranberries. Line a baking sheet with wax paper.

2. Over very low heat, melt 3 ounces of the dark chocolate in the top part of a double boiler (the water should be simmering slightly) and stir frequently. (Note: the water should not be touching the top pan).

3. Remove the double boiler from the heat and stir in the rest of the chocolate. Remove the top pan with the chocolate in it and set it aside.

4. Replace the simmering water in the bottom pan with warm tap water; put the pan of melted chocolate on top of the warm water to keep the chocolate at the right temperature while you make the clusters.

5. Stir the fruit-nut mixture into the chocolate. Spoon out tablespoon-sized clusters of the chocolate mixture onto the baking sheet, about an inch apart. Put them in the refrigerator to set for about 15 minutes. Store/serve at room temperature.

Tip: If you do not have a double boiler, you can improvise with a saucepan and bowl.

Chapter 4

Fat Mess vs. Hot Dress: You Decide

Making That Little Black Dress Fit

You've got the most fabulous dress. Unfortunately, you have one of two major problems. Number one, it doesn't zip despite the sucking in and the three people holding it in place and the fourth one doing the zipping (a common occurrence). Number two, you can get it on your body but it resembles a sausage casing. I've experienced both dilemmas. Listen to this one: weeks before a close friend's wedding I could only stare at, but not wear, the gorgeous, every girl's dream, endlessly desired Vera Wang bridesmaid dress hanging ever so perfectly in my closet. I hate to make excuses for the extra layer of fat on my ass that week, but believe me when I say my reasons were valid. Blame Marcus Samuelsson for making me lunch that week, Missy Robbins for feeding me pasta with enough butter and oil to provide my body with its own insulation layer, John DeLucie for crafting the perfect chicken pot pie for me at the Waverly Inn, and, last but not least, Todd English for teaching me how to make homemade mozzarella at the Mohegan Sun in Connecticut. Come on, who could resist all of that? Whoever the culprit, the result was still the same. I was a pork chop, and despite my experience at being a bridesmaid (circa twenty-five times), I was fresh out of ideas. We've all been there before—late nights at the office, too much stress, too much good, free food available, which all ends up taking residence on your thighs. There are always times when that special occasion is coming up and you have to get fit in a flash. For these occasions, I tap into Behind the Burner's network of nutritionists and food mood doctors, some skinny girlfriends, and voilà . . . I get back on track so I can make it out of the dressing room alive.

Fad diets = Fad do-nots. Most girls' first inclination is heading to the vitamin store for some pills or the bookstore for the next weight loss manual. DON'T DO EITHER! Both will screw up your system, including your metabolic rate and will cause you to lose pounds that you can't keep off. Fad diets and drugstore supplements are only for short-term gain and long-term pain (and damage). I believe in tough love. You're gonna do this the hard way—the way I do it. It works for me, so it should work for you.

Start by writing down what you eat. The power of the pen will reveal all the crap that is entering your holy temple (your body). You will be reluctant to admit the donuts you eat with your cream-saturated latte, or that massive slice of cheesecake you had for dessert that was just "heavenly." Sex is heavenly, cheesecake is not. Being forced to write foolish, "had to have" treats that are pure sugar and fat in your mouth is just embarrassing. Seeing is believing! You'll be more inclined to pass them over to your friends, secretly wishing that poor life decision will show up on their tummies tomorrow while yours stays flat as a pancake.

Lay off the booze, all you party people. I am not crazy; I am not saying you can't have a good time, but you must be mindful before flirting with the bartender two weeks before your big event. Loading up on alcoholic drinks is just a recipe for piling up empty calories. In addition, just like the beer goggles that caused you to end up with Mr. Unibrow, alcohol can cloud your judgment and make you lose your mojo and inspiration to eat healthy. Besides, once you're in that dress for the evening, you can booze (one glass of red wine, please!)—it's worth the wait. I manage to be pretty good in this department, opting for soda water and a splash of cranberry when I'm out. Caffeine is also a no-no, it increases appetite and cravings, so just because you're avoiding margaritas and mojitos don't think having four Cokes in one night is being an angel. Here are three reasons why I haven't drunk Coke since I enjoyed it with a piece of cheese pizza in high school: 1. It's sugar. It rots your teeth and depletes calcium from your bones. Ew! Sorry, but I don't want to be a rotting corpse till I'm actually in the grave. 2. The calories, need I say more? 3. It's all chemicals. While trying to get into that dress, your mind-set needs to change. If it doesn't grow in the ground or on the trees, it shouldn't go in your mouth. Stick to the pure stuff. No ifs, ands, or buts.

Abandon desserts. While these are my true weakness, I steer clear of all sweets when gearing up for a big event. The sugar, the fat, and the calories will all find a home on your belly. Now, do we really want to look pregnant all year round? Every time I get the urge for something sweet, I snack on some berries and add honey, or have a small piece of dark chocolate because it is filled with flavonols and antioxidants. One of the perks of my job is getting gourmet food samples all the time. I keep a stash of dark chocolate (65 percent cacao and up) in our office kitchen cabinet at work at all times in case my female hormones get hold of me. Dried fruit can have a lot of sugar, but it's better after dinner than chocolate mousse. Don't be afraid of a few dried cherries, apricots, or cranberries.

Don't miss a meal. Every meal counts and keeps your body's metabolism running. Eating a few small meals a day instead of three big ones is ideal. If you feel hungry in between, opt for healthy snacks like string cheese, a few almonds, or a tablespoon of nut butter. The protein in these snacks will tide you over to your next meal.

Channel your inner chef. Getting fit and fabulous is about feeling good on the inside and looking good on the outside. Start by throwing out all that processed crap you have at home. Anything with more chemicals in the ingredients list (ones you can't pronounce, no less) than natural ingredients should be abandoned. Yes, Pop-Tarts deserve to sit in your garbage, as well as that Easy Mac crap, potato chips (I don't care if they're baked), and the cookie stash you hide from everyone but yourself. It's time to stop looking and get cooking. Plan on making yourself breakfast, lunch, and dinner. Okay, maybe that's a bit ambitious, but even two out of three meals made by you will make a HUGE difference on your waistline. Bountiful breakfasts (see Chapter 5, Eating Muffins Gives You Muffin Top), lean lunches, and delectable dinners that are fueled up with protein, fresh fruits, and vegetables will get you ready to rock that dress.

Sodium is sinful. It makes your stomach expand like the

Goodyear blimp. Sodium clings to water and gives you that oh so bloated look and feel. So resist your craving for munching on salted nuts, don't reach for that second helping of soy sauce, and absolutely no potato chips should touch your lips! Follow these rules and reduce your sodium intake; you will feel the water weight falling right off your body.

Speaking of water, drink as much as possible. Eight glasses are ideal—about four 16-ounce water bottles per day. Make them tasty with lime, lemon, cinnamon, or cucumber slices (the silica is also good for your skin). Water will help flush out the toxins in your body and get your belly red-carpet-ready.

Take vitamins. We all know you took the Flintstones ones as a child. So why'd you stop? March your ass to the closest pharmacy and make your purchase. Try to eat foods with natural nutrients, but a little extra vitamin C and E on top of that will make your skin look great. For some reason, vitamins, like drinking lots of water and eating fiber, make me poop—the highlight of my day, and yet another reason to fill up your medicine cabinet.

Say good-bye to "bad" carbs, not all carbs. When I overload on carbs—risotto is just too inviting to resist on a winter day—my belly develops a distinct Oompa Loompa bulge. Sugars, white flour, white bread, and all other white stuff (no, I am not being racist here), should be banished while you're trying your best to get into your dress. I'm not an Atkins follower, so I never cut out carbs completely, even if I have a wardrobe fantasy that would inspire me to do so. The Atkins diet actually restricts healthful complex carbs in vegetables and fruits that are known to protect against heart disease. I think it is just impractical living. Instead, I stick to whole grains and try to have them for lunch or breakfast instead of for dinner.

Fiber is your friend. My old boss's assistant introduced me to Colonics. It seemed like a hocus-pocus powder that made me poop like a banshee. After a week of having it every day, I had essentially crapped out everything in my body right down to the fried foods I ate before *Beverly Hills 90210* (the first season) went on the air. Something about it felt unnatural, so I decided to naturalize the process by eating fiber in its raw form and only while still getting the same effect. Before a big event, I load up on fiber-rich foods (apples, berries, broccoli, spinach, Brussels sprouts, kale, green beans, nuts, rye, whole wheat, etc.), and let Mother Nature work her magic. I used to make fun of my chronically constipated mother sprinkling bran all over her fish, but now I know why. Apparently it runs in the family. I discovered an age-old Indian remedy, called Isabgol, essentially psyllium husk (which can be purchased at your local Indian market). You take one teaspoon at night with a big glass of water and come sunshine, your natural detox will have arrived. I follow this routine during fashion week just to chase away the twinge of jealousy I feel when I see superskinny models strutting down the runway in the latest fashions. Still, I'm proud I'm not them—I LOVE to eat!

No late-night leftovers. Trust me, you're really not as hungry as you think. After a late day glued to my computer at work or a marathon of events in one night, I come home and immediately want to raid my cupboard. After high stress or high levels of activity, I crave comfort food. It's not even about hunger. It's about feeling gratification from a greasy spoon before crawling into bed. Avoid the greasy spoon, and you can engage with the pillow a lot faster and dream about the food. Seems like a good deal to me. If you want to be the bridesmaid that is holding her dress together with a slew of safety pins, then don't listen to me. If you don't, try to cut off your food intake after 9:00 P.M. (or earlier, depending on how late you go to sleep).

Workouts work wonders. For all of you quant jocks, figure this one out: calories in − calories out = inches padding your jelly belly. Simply said, get moving. Walk, run, bike, kickbox, do sit-ups, take those crazy Pilates classes that all the high-class house-wives rave about and get your body into gear. Lift some weights while you're at it to double the impact with strength training. I amp up my workouts before photo ops, as I feel like they kick me up a notch. Not to mention they make my skin look radiant and I sleep better at night. But beware, excessive exercise is dangerous. Tread with caution. I am in no way instructing you to become a gym-obsessed muscle maniac. And, quite frankly, I get hun-grier and eat more when I exercise, so it is even more important to make healthy choices when you're breaking a sweat.

So ditch the thought of buying overpriced Spanx. I've never gone down that road and never plan to. Fit your slim body into that dress the healthy way. If you don't, you're only cheating yourself, and that's just sad! Besides, rock-star dresses deserve rock-star bodies with true talent. You want to look your best among the usual crowd of scantily clad leggy models and media moguls behaving badly. Do it the healthy way. No fake anorexic pill-obsessed divas welcome.

Five Ways to Limit Your Calorie Intake During a Night Out

Let's be honest: muffin top doesn't look good with anything hanging in your closet. So it's important to plan your meals ac-cordingly before a big night out on the town. Here's a quick recap of the things you can do to cut calories and avoid the 4:00 a.m. munchies during girls' night out.

1. *Eat before you go.* This is especially true for events like weddings, where a waiter carrying a full tray of cheese puffs seems to be lurking around every corner. Come hungry but not famished. Free food usually equals an excuse to pig out, but it doesn't have to.

2. *Avoid the late-night munchies.* Although hitting the local pizza joint at all hours of the night may have been the rage in college, try to leave those habits behind. Eating late-night pizza and fried food is almost guaranteeing weight gain overnight. Instead, go straight to bed after a long night out and save your appetite for a hearty breakfast in the morning. Trust me, you won't starve to death at 3:00 a.m.

3. *Drink up, take in less.* By now, most of us know to avoid those Long Island iced teas, which might as well be called Fat Island iced teas. But a cranberry and vodka doesn't exactly cut calories either. Avoid the sugary juices and stick to tonic water as a mixer, or low-calorie beer or wine when enjoying a few drinks. Whatever you do, don't order one of those margaritas that comes in a glass the size of your head.

4. *Taste tester.* Rather than starve yourself at large events or fun dinners, indulge and taste a bit of everything. If you're eating out, suggest splitting an appetizer with someone and order one dessert for the table, so that everyone can have a taste without the caloric aftermath. If you're at an event with

a buffet, try sampling a bit of everything—just limit your taste-testing to one taste per dish, please.

5. *Drink water between each alcoholic drink.* Aside from the benefit of avoiding a deadly hangover, drinking water between each drink keeps you stay fuller longer and controls the amount of alcohol you put down in one night. It also keeps you hydrated on the dance floor. Remember, overdrinking is just as bad as, if not worse than, overeating, especially if you are trying to lose weight. Alcohol will always be your biggest setback from achieving this goal, so don't forget to order that agua after every drink!

THINGS
YOUR
DOCTOR
WON'T
TELL YOU

Chapter 5

Eating Muffins Gives You Muffin Top

A Healthy Breakfast Is a Must for My Firm Ass and Bust

I can still hear my mom's voice screeching in my head, "Eat your breakfast before you get on the bus!" Last night's left-over Domino's Pizza? I don't think so. My mother was a junk food Nazi. Only healthy cereals were allowed in our house. You know, the kinds that looked and tasted like cardboard. I was permitted to mix Kix with Total and that's how I'd get my wannabe sugar fix. I was a cereal addict and often traded in a bowl of spaghetti and meatballs for Banana Nut Crunch with two percent milk for dinner.

Truth be told, Mom was right. The cliché that eating breakfast is a must rings true and is even more pertinent today. The first meal of the day fuels your brain. It's the gas that gets us going and helps us tackle and cope with the world. And believe me, there's been a lot to deal with: third-grade multiplication tables, college chemistry, financial modeling at Goldman Sachs, board meetings as a venture capitalist, and filming TV segments at Behind the Burner. Trust me—life only gets more complicated as you get older, so start simple and fill your car up with the premium stuff. Garbage (sugar, sodium, empty calories) will not get you very far.

As the years have passed, I've been through many cycles of breakfast favorites. After the cereal addiction, there was the bagel phase (with low-fat cream cheese because I was convinced I was being "oh so healthy"), muffin madness, and French toast frenzy. I never skipped breakfast since my grumbling stomach would not allow me, but I often made the unhealthiest choices possible. Working crazy hours with a career in finance and now even crazier hours with a career in media, breakfast was always on-the-go. Egg and cheese sandwiches on a white roll from my local deli were a Friday guilty pleasure. Until I got fat, and then I got smart so I could get UN-fat. Who would have known eating muffins gives you muffin top?

Rise and shine! You've just spent the last eight hours sleeping. Every day, you roll out of bed, completely dehydrated, and you've got one thing on your mind, "How am I going to get to [work, school, daycare] on time?" You rush through your somewhat nonexistent beauty routine and head out the door. Did you make your bed before you locked your door? Who cares! Breakfast is an afterthought and takes its form in a comforting flaky croissant during your commute, cup of coffee, or a cigarette while you're stuck in traffic or waiting for the train. The problem is, carb-laden treats, caffeine, or nicotine have you thinking about lunch at 10:00 A.M. on the dot. A lack of protein fails to satiate while sugar and caffeine give your blood sugar spikes and lows, yielding a craving for more food and sugar. So, let's restart this one the right way . . .

What I discovered is that there is no easy way out. Yo-yo diets will have you bouncing from Kate Beckinsale to Kirstie Alley in no time. The only way to win this game is to make small yet permanent changes to your lifestyle. From making better choices at breakfast to cutting just 100 to 200 calories out of your daily garbage-filled diet, you will see results OVER TIME (be patient!). The weight may come off slowly or not at all (muscle weighs more than fat), but the leaner, lovelier you won't just be making a cameo. She'll be here to stay.

#1 DRINK WATER. Start your day off with a glass of H_2O. It will help flush out the toxins and fill you up so you don't crave a crappy breakfast.

#2 NEVER SKIP BREAKFAST. Your body will hate you and missing breakfast will manifest itself later in evil ways. You think you don't need it, but you do. Mamma knows best, so obey her command in your head. Not eating breakfast will make you hungrier for lunch and result in weight GAIN, not loss. If you skip "the most important meal of the day" you will end up with low sugar levels all morning and you'll end up craving sugar and making the wrong choices for lunch.

#3 MAKE YOUR OWN BREAKFAST WHEN PRACTICALLY POSSIBLE. As they say, what you see is what you get . . . so therefore, when you don't see it, you don't know what you are getting. Your egg white omelet could be cooked in enough oil to fry a chicken (YIKES!). As a chef, I've worked in restaurant kitchens and I simply love restaurant dining. But, truth be told, breakfast is not the meal to ingest all those calories. It's a waste because you're not even getting a good glass of Tempranillo with it. Chefs make food that tastes good. Butter is not an ingredient; it's a tool to achieve a particular outcome. Those crispy home fries that hit the spot have bacon fat that you might as well staple to your ass.

Take matters into your own hands. Boil eggs while you're getting ready and take them with you so you can eat them at school or work. Pack yogurt to eat at your desk. Greek yogurt is my favorite because it packs in a protein punch. Sprinkle it with roasted flax seeds and you've got a spa breakfast. A girl needs her sweets, so I add honey instead of jam or slices of ripe banana. Go tropical and throw in some berries for some added color, nutrients, flavor, and texture. Trust me, it is not a fad—you will be glad. I load up on raspberries, blueberries, and blackberries, which are teeming with antioxidants (to fight those wrinkles that haven't quite shown up yet) and rich in fiber. Almonds sprinkled in yogurt give it a good crunch and nutrients like fiber and vitamin E. Sometimes I whip up an egg white omelet (I skip the yolks for less fat and cholesterol) with lots of colorful veggies like spinach and red peppers. Adding a red pepper will give me the vitamin C I need for a whole day (again I'm taking preventive measures for those wrinkles that are imminent). Other days, I'll spread almond butter on whole-grain toast or a rice cake. When it comes to breakfast carbs, keep in mind: brown is beautiful and always better for you.

When I'm really in a rush, like many of us are, I make myself a smoothie, take it and go. Simply throw into a blender: fruit of your choice, low-fat or soymilk (extra protein), and ice or frozen yogurt. The great thing about smoothies is that they're so versatile and can be made as a midday snack. Try bananas, vanilla soymilk, ice, and vanilla extract for a faux-dessert, or take a cue from Gwyneth Paltrow and use almond milk instead, and an extra nutritional dose of ProGreen's probiotic powder. I stay away from powders but my pals, a.k.a. the diet divas, seem to like them.

Protein and fiber are your breakfast buddies. Lean meat, eggs, beans, and low-fat dairy satiate and give you the protein that will hold you over till lunch, or in my case, till your midmorning snack. Fiber is equally important and gets that morning toilet bowl flushing. So stock your fridge and get some grains, veggies, and fruits in your system. If you spent last night chasing down cocktails, you need water more than you know. That headache is probably from dehydration and H_2O is the only remedy. Pill popping (besides painkillers, but I just don't bother with that stuff) is for anorexic tennis moms who are in denial about their plastic surgery. There's a natural solution to every man-made problem, so always try that first. Water should be your beverage of choice not only for breakfast, but for every meal. Sugary juices will give you a high, followed by a big crash. I don't touch coffee (only like the flavor when I'm licking it off an ice cream cone) and drink antioxidant-filled green tea (gotta love the immune system booster!) on rare occasions. I know this will make my sister sad, but coffee's high dose of caffeine not only sends you on the high-and-low roller coaster, but also creates an addiction. To me, addictions are a sign of weakness. I am strong, not weak. Hence, I let my co-workers enjoy the fancy Nescafé coffee machine while I drink water with a slice of lemon or a sprinkle of cinnamon if I'm feeling fancy.

I must admit I am a miserable person and essentially an inanimate object before I eat breakfast. I usually get to bed pretty late, so I wake up on empty, needing a real jump start to my day.

Eating breakfast speeds up my metabolism, makes me alert, and gives me the energy I need to dodge bike messengers on my morning walk to the office. I literally can't think straight until I've eaten. This important meal gave me the ability to focus at school (Look, Ma, straight A's!) and now lets me power through meetings and high-stress mornings at work.

Oh, and if you are not hungry in the morning, do breakfast anyway. Even those probiotic yogurt drinks count. Grab an apple or banana and you are on your way. Remember what they say: even an apple a day can keep the doctor away. Your blood sugar levels will thank you later.

411 on Caffeine

I'm not really a coffee drinker. To me there's no real point in starting my day off bitter and dark like the brew I'm sipping. Instead, I resort to green tea that has the antioxidants I need to boost me up without weighing me down. This is not to say that caffeine is terrible for you; in moderate doses it can keep you running around the office, but overdosing on this drug-like substance can have visceral effects. Below are a few things you may not know about caffeine:

1. Caffeine is found in sixty different types of plants around the world, including but not limited to cocoa beans, coffee beans, tea leaves, and kola nuts. Any excuse for a bite of dark chocolate is okay with me!

2. Despite rumors, caffeine does not cause the following: cancer, rapid increase in blood pressure, stroke, or heart disease. In moderate amounts (think two to three cups of coffee a day), caffeine can improve performance and keep up energy levels,

according to the American Cancer Society.

3. On the downside, more than six cups can lead to nervousness, sweating, tension, upset stomach, anxiety, and even more unattractive traits we don't usually want people to know we have.

4. Caffeine is mildly addictive. Used moderately, it poses no health risk, but if you decide to quit cold turkey, you may experience headaches, fatigue, irritability, and depression. I suggest gradual weaning to avoid most of these symptoms, just as I would, for say, cigarette smoking.

Here's a rundown of the average amounts of caffeine found in most coffee, soda, and tea beverages:

Instant coffeee: 75 mg
Brewed coffee: 85 mg
Brewed tea: 50 mg
Energy drinks: 28–87 mg
Soda: 24 mg
Chocolate: 5.5–35.5 mg
(Source: faqs.org/nutrition)

If you have to get your caffeine fix, I'd go with green tea as your drug of choice. It contains antioxidants that can help prevent cancer, and it has been proven to boost metabolism. Drink green tea iced or with a splash of honey. Whatever you do, it'll be healthier for you by reducing food cravings, lowering cholesterol, and preventing tooth decay (I know, right?).

Muffins That Won't Give You Muffin Top

MAKES 12 MUFFINS

1 cup rolled oats
1 cup low fat milk
1 cup whole wheat flour
1 teaspoon baking powder
½ teaspoon baking soda
1 teaspoon cinnamon
1 teaspoon flax seed
1 teaspoon salt
½ cup brown sugar
½ cup applesauce
1 egg
1 teaspoon vanilla extract

This muffin will give you fiber instead of loads of fat to keep you full.

Nutrition Facts

Amount Per Serving		
Calories 112		
Total Fat 1.2g		
Trans Fat 0.0g		
Cholesterol 17mg		
Sodium 263mg		
Total Carbohydrates 22.3g		
Dietary Fiber 1.4g		
Sugars 9.1g		
Protein 3.2g		
Vitamin A 1%	•	Vitamin C 0%
Calcium 6%	•	Iron 5%

1. Preheat your oven to 375° F. Grease 12 muffin cups or line with paper muffin liners.

2. Pour the milk over the oats in a small bowl. Let sit while you are mixing the other ingredients.

3. Stir together the whole wheat flour, baking powder, baking soda, cinnamon, flax seed, salt, and brown sugar in a large mixing bowl. Stir in the milk and oat mixture, applesauce, egg, and vanilla; and mix it all together. Pour the batter into the prepared muffin cups.

4. Bake in a preheated oven for 30 minutes, or until a toothpick inserted into the center of a muffin comes out clean. Check the muffins after 20 minutes, as your oven may cook them faster than other standard ovens.

Tip: Make the batter the night before, refrigerate it, and bake the muffins in the morning.

Strawberry Banana Breakfast Smoothie

MAKES 1 SERVING

½ cup nonfat milk
½ cup fat-free plain yogurt
½ fresh banana,
    peeled and chopped
1½ tablespoons flax seed
1 teaspoon honey
½ cup fresh strawberries

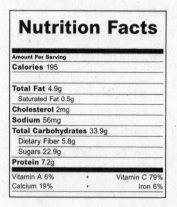

Nutrition Facts		
Amount Per Serving		
Calories 195		
Total Fat 4.9g		
Saturated Fat 0.5g		
Cholesterol 2mg		
Sodium 56mg		
Total Carbohydrates 33.9g		
Dietary Fiber 5.8g		
Sugars 22.9g		
Protein 7.2g		
Vitamin A 6%	•	Vitamin C 79%
Calcium 19%	•	Iron 6%

1. In a blender, combine the milk, yogurt, banana, flax seed, honey, and strawberries and blend until smooth.

2. Pour into a glass and enjoy.

Tip: Strawberries are the first fruit to ripen in the spring. The best bananas for eating are those that are a solid yellow color specked with brown.

Frittata Mexican Style

½ cup chopped green peppers
½ cup chopped onions
½ cup chopped mushrooms
1 tablespoon olive oil
4 tablespoons salsa
4 large eggs
2 tablespoons low-fat milk
½ cup shredded Cheddar cheese

Nutrition Facts	
Amount Per Serving	
Calories 176	
Total Fat 13.2g	
Saturated Fat 5.1g	
Cholesterol 227mg	
Sodium 259mg	
Total Carbohydrates 4.1g	
Dietary Fiber 0.8g	
Sugars 2.4g	
Protein 10.8g	
Vitamin A 10%	Vitamin C 18%
Calcium 15%	Iron 7%

1. Preheat your oven to 350° F.

2. Sauté the vegetables in olive oil, then add the salsa and reduce for 2 minutes.

3. While the vegetable and salsa mixture is reducing, take a mixing bowl and add the eggs and low-fat milk. Mix gently.

4. Pour the egg and milk mixture into the veggies and cook for 2 minutes.

5. Sprinkle the cheese on top and place the sauté pan (make sure it doesn't have a plastic handle) in the oven.

6. Bake for 20 to 25 minutes, or until a knife is clear after cutting through the center.

Tip: When sautéing vegetables, cut them all approximately the same size for even cooking time.

Strawberry Go Nuts Smoothie

MAKES 1 SERVING

5 frozen whole strawberries
½ cup low-fat milk or almond milk
¼ cup (2 ounces) silken tofu
1 tablespoon brown sugar

1. Combine the strawberries, milk, tofu, and sugar in a blender and blend for about a minute (until the mixture is frothy and smooth).

2. Pour into a glass and enjoy.

Tip: Almond milk is lower in fat than skim or low-fat milk and adds delicious flavor.

Nutrition Facts		
Amount Per Serving		
Calories 144		
Total Fat 3.7g		
Saturated Fat 1.3g		
Cholesterol 6mg		
Sodium 64mg		
Total Carbohydrates 20.5g		
Dietary Fiber 1.7g		
Sugars 18.3g		
Protein 9.2g		
Vitamin A 5%	•	Vitamin C 59%
Calcium 28%	•	Iron 7%

Chapter 6

Supersize It

These Superfoods Keep Me Looking
and Feeling Like Wonder Woman

Ask ten nutritionists which superfoods you should eat and they
will give you 10 different answers. They will, however, agree
that every girl has got to get her superfoods (without supersiz-
ing herself, of course). Whether it's to prevent cancer or to ward
off heart disease, consuming these power sources will move
you forward a long way on the race to good health. I've learned
amazing facts and figures from the renowned nutritionists who
work with Behind the Burner. Also, my mom has been reading
Jane E. Brody's Personal Health column in the *New York Times*
and e-mailing me links to the articles since e-mail was invented.
Mom is convinced that superfoods will help her live as long as
a Chinese grandmother. Don't hate the Chinese women, who
seem to make it to their nineties with beauty and grace. Just try

to be like them. Are you ready for the amazing impact of my favorite superfoods? Eat your heart out.

Blueberries Keep Your Belly in Check

Packed with vitamins A, B complex, C, E, and antioxidants, these delicious berries can lower your risk of heart disease and cancer while boosting up your immune system. Better yet, a University of Michigan cardiovascular study suggests that blueberries may help reduce belly fat. Don't you want to say goodbye to all the elastic waistbands in your closet?

How I Enjoy Them

In a smoothie, over multigrain cereal, with Greek yogurt and honey, over a multigrain waffle for breakfast, alone as an afternoon snack, sprinkled with a little brown sugar or tossed over frozen yogurt for dessert. Try to efface those memories of blueberry blintzes and accept your mortality. Blueberries can also be tossed into buckwheat pancakes. Get inventive, people!

Avocados for All Occasions

Recent research has demonstrated that avocados also offer some surprising and powerful health benefits. Sure, they're high in fat, but avocados contain what is known as monounsaturated fat, or a healthy form of fat, not to mention a great oxymoron for you grammar lovers. Monounsaturated fat is linked to a reduced risk of cancer, heart disease, and diabetes. The monounsaturated fat in avocados comes from oleic acid, which may also help lower cholesterol.

Avocados are loaded with 9 to 17 grams of fiber and are a good source of lutein, an antioxidant linked to eye and skin health. Who knew beauty could be delicious? They top the charts among all fruits for folate, potassium, vitamin E, and magnesium. Indeed, the very impressive health benefits of eating avocados regularly have encouraged me to adopt them as a new superfood.

There are generally two types of avocados available in U.S. markets—the California Hass avocado and the Florida West Indian avocado. Hass avocados are nutty and buttery and rich in healthy monounsaturated oil—ranging from 18 to 30 percent oil in each avocado. The light green Florida avocado is larger and juicier than the Hass variety, but it is less buttery and considerably lower in oil. I prefer the West Coast option; however, the Florida avocado contains just 3 to 5 percent oil and roughly 25 to 50 percent less fat than the Hass type.

How I Enjoy Them

Envision those beach babes in Laguna. Picture those Malibu bikinis and all that California has to offer. I know gals who make tuna salad with avocado; or one of my nephew's favorites: added on top of an omelet. Other ways to partake: diced up in a salad, sliced with turkey in a sandwich or burger bun, or mashed in a dip. My favorite, however, is guacamole. Enjoy the taste of Mexico all year round by slicing the avocado vertically and adding freshly diced tomatoes, cilantro, and onions for the perfect snack. Remember to always keep the pit of the avocado in the guacamole so it doesn't turn brown.

Apples to Apples

An apple a day really does keep the doctor away. Here's why:

Apples are loaded with antioxidants and fiber, which protect cells from damage, reducing the risk of cancer and cardiovascular disease, especially if you eat the skin. Past studies prove that apples help prevent breast cancer, liver cancer, and diabetes.

Think only milk is good for your bones? Wrong! Apples include the mineral boron, which helps strengthen bones (up to 2.7 mg/kg). French researchers found that a flavonoid called phloridzin that is found only in apples increases bone density and may protect menopausal women from osteoporosis.

The pectin in apples lowers LDL ("bad") cholesterol. People who eat two apples per day may lower their cholesterol by as much as 16 percent. Besides, you should always eat two fruits a day to speed up your metabolism.

Not a friend of fruit? Apple juice is beneficial too. Studies show that children with asthma who drink more apple juice suffer from less wheezing than children who hardly drink it. I prefer Mott's apple juice, hands down. There is Mott's for Tots available now too; less sugar makes the mommies happy.

How I Enjoy Them

Snacking on apples on the go couldn't have been made easier. No cheese platter is complete without one. Or slice the apple and coat it with almond or natural peanut butter; eat it alone, or with chicken or pork in a sauce; baked in an apple crisp as a dessert. Apple butter is a good substitute for butter or margarine on toast. And it's only 35 calories per serving.

Fish for the Soul

Health wise, fish makes for the perfect dish. Eating fish helps cut the risk of heart disease, cancer, Alzheimer's, stroke, diabetes, and arthritis. The American Heart Association recommends that adults eat at least two fish meals per week, especially wild salmon, herring, and sardines (they're great on pizza!), because those varieties provide the most heart-healthy omega-3 fatty acids. Avoid fish containing high amounts of mercury—

and not just when you're pregnant. Steer the boat clear of shark (I thought *they* ate *us*?), swordfish, tilefish, and marlin.

Other forms of omega-3's are available in fortified eggs, flax seed, and walnuts. These superfoods have the added benefit of being high in monounsaturated fats, which can lower cholesterol.

How I Enjoy It

Call it kiddie but lightly sautéed fish with garlic paired with haricot verts is my favorite. Also enjoyable is sashimi, tuna in a salad, tuna with celery (skip the mayo unless you're using a little Smart Balance with Omega-3) in a sandwich, or marinated salmon, grilled or baked for dinner with a side of veggies. Baked haddock sprinkled with garlic and herbs is another favorite. Shellfish such as steamed clams and mussels are low in fat and high in protein. Most think that because mussels are high in flesh cholesterol, they increase human cholesterol. This is false.

Although not the healthiest choice in the sea, baked clams are to die for—stuffed with bread crumbs seasoned with parsley, garlic, onion, basil, salt, and pepper, and drizzled with freshly squeezed lemon juice, they are a personal favorite.

Garlic Attack

This bulb may prevent some hard-core lip action, but it definitely prevails when it comes to your health. Research shows that garlic lowers total cholesterol and triglyceride (blood fat) levels, helping prevent clogged arteries. Compounds in garlic have been shown to stop the spread of both skin and prostate cancer. A compound in garlic called ajoene is a natural antioxidant that has anticlotting abilities, thus helping in the prevention of heart disease and strokes. It has even been shown to be an effective antifungal agent for treating yeast infections, vaginitis, and athlete's foot. Bye-bye Monistat creams.

Here's a fun fact for cooks: Research has shown that cooking garlic with meat reduces carcinogenic chemicals (now that's a tongue twister) in cooked meat that are believed to be linked to breast cancer for women. Garlic has been shown to reduce inflammation and pain in the body for those suffering from osteoarthritis and rheumatoid arthritis. Forget antibiotics and over-the-counter overpriced crap that never works—keep it natural like the old days. Garlic serves as a remedy for the cold and flu. Because of its antiviral and antibacterial properties as well as its vitamin C content, garlic serves as a powerful agent against these illnesses. Every single time I feel a sore throat or cold coming on, I reach for a few cloves of garlic and suck on them. I'd rather be stinky and sweating garlic than be sick! Can't stand garlic breath? If you can't tolerate a Listerine strip that will burn your tongue, chew on a sprig of parsley.

How I Enjoy It

In anything and everything, I LOVE garlic. From sucking on it raw when I'm sick to cooking with it, I make garlic part of my everyday eating. Where do we begin? Roast it in the oven and mix into butter and dried herbs for sensational garlic bread. Sauté it in olive oil and toss in blanched broccoli, fresh spinach, or asparagus for a tasty side dish. Dress boiled pasta with minced, browned garlic and add sausage and sun-dried tomatoes. Marinate any proteins with raw slices of garlic for an earthy special flavor. Garlic is a global concept. Get with it.

Mushrooms as Medicine

Mushrooms have been used in Eastern medicine for centuries. They have powerful effects on the immune system—especially the maitake, shiitake, and reishi varieties. Mushrooms are used as a form of cancer treatment throughout Asia because of their ability to counteract the toxic effects of chemotherapy and radiation while also shrinking tumors. Japanese researchers have found that regularly eating shiitake mushrooms lowers blood cholesterol levels up to 45 percent.

Mushrooms are an excellent source of potassium. One medium portobello mushroom has even more potassium than a banana. One serving of mushrooms also provides about 20 to 40 percent of the daily value of copper, a mineral that has cardioprotective properties.

Shiitake mushrooms have been used for centuries by the Chinese and Japanese to treat colds and the flu. Lentinan, a betaglucan isolated from the fruiting body of shiitake mushrooms, appears to stimulate the immune system, help fight infection, and demonstrates antitumor activity.

How I Enjoy Them

Wipe off any dirt with a moist cloth and slice into salads or bake in a frittata. Sauté in balsamic vinegar and onions or stuff with goat cheese and bake. Sauté with olive oil and garlic, or sauté with soy sauce and sesame oil. Even whole wheat pasta is pleasurable with mushrooms and chicken in a white wine sauce.

Eggstatic about Eggs

The queen of protein is the egg. Aside from containing all nine essential amino acids, eggs are loaded with nutrients. Eggs are also great for the eyes. An egg a day may help prevent macular degeneration. For God's sake, don't be afraid to eat the yolks. I eat them about twice a week and go for whites the rest of the week. For all those who obsess over egg white omelets, egg yolks actually contain choline, which helps protect heart and brain function and prevents cholesterol and fat from accumulating in the liver. New research shows that moderate consumption of eggs is not harmful for cholesterol levels. In fact, recent studies have shown that regular consumption of two eggs per day does not affect a person's lipid profile and may even improve it.

One egg contains just 5 grams of fat and only 1.5 grams of that is saturated fat. Listen up, ladies: eggs also promote healthy hair and nails because of their high sulfur content. Beauty comes from the inside out. Eggs may even prevent breast cancer. In one study, women who consumed at least six eggs a week lowered their risk of breast cancer by 44 percent.

How I Enjoy Them

I think I was born with an egg in my mouth. It's been a journey from egg salad sandwiches in my Barbie lunchbox to an integral part of my daily breakfast routine. Sunny-side up with whole-grain English muffins, hard boiled with a teaspoon of vinegar (trust me, it's delicious), in an omelet packed with veggies, or sliced over salad. I also love egg drop soup, one of the few healthy options on a Chinese takeout menu.

Uncover the Mystery Behind Flax Seeds

Most people underestimate the power of the seed. Gandhi himself proclaimed, "Wherever flax seed becomes a regular food item among the people, there will be better health."

Recent studies have suggested that flax seed may protect against cancer, particularly breast cancer, prostate cancer, and colon cancer. Remember to grind your flax seeds to maximize the health benefits and be sure to keep them refrigerated. In animal studies, the plant omega-3 fatty acid found in flax seed, called ALA, inhibited tumor incidence and growth. Second, the lignans (estrogenlike chemicals that act as antioxidants) in flax seed may provide some protection against cancers that are sensitive to hormones.

How I Enjoy It

Toss your chicken or veal Milanese in it—then bake or sauté. Lip-smacking good for you and your dinner guests. I add flax seed to fruit smoothies and to my oatmeal (after it is cooked). Flax seed loses its value upon heating, so always add flax seed to cooled substances. When eating flax seed straight, chew thoroughly and follow it by a big glass of water. Also, sprinkle it in your morning yogurt or cottage cheese.

Red Wine and Dine

Wine is not just a staple of candlelit Valentine's Day dinners. A glass of red wine can be enjoyed each day to increase HDL cholesterol and reduce the risk of blood clots. Red wine also contains powerful antioxidants, which may help your cardiovascular system. But don't get carried away at the dinner table; more than one drink daily has been linked to high blood pressure. Sip mindfully and chillax.

How I Enjoy It

Red wine is always my drink of choice. Give me a glass of Pinot Noir, Montepulciano, or Layer Cake Malbec and I'm singing a happy tune. I also use red wine to make sauces for meats, seafood, and pasta. Imagine a garlicky ground-turkey Bolognese reduced in red wine and coated with an aged Parmigiano. Not bad at all.

Cinnamon

Not only does cinnamon add a warm, spicy flavor to both sweet and savory dishes, but the antioxidants in one teaspoon of cinnamon equal those in a full cup of pomegranate juice. Cinnamon also contains significant amounts of polyphenols, which keep blood sugar levels under control.

How I Enjoy It

I add a bit to my morning coffee for extra flavor, sprinkle it in yogurt for a spicy kick, or throw a dash of it on fruit salads. And nothing complements apples like spicy cinnamon, so feel free to use a heavy hand when making applesauce or my fabulous baked apples (see page TK).

Parmesan Cheese

If you want strong bones that will carry you into old age, start loading up on all the calcium you can get. Yogurt and lowfat milk are great sources of calcium and vitamins, but who wants to consume 3 servings a day? Instead, try sneaking more Parmesan cheese into your diet. With 340 mg of calcium per ounce (as compared to about 200 mg in Swiss cheese), you'll be on the fast track to reaching the recommended 1000 mg per day.

How I Enjoy It

A small shaving of Parmesan goes a long way as a topping for pasta or vegetable dishes. I also like to sprinkle a bit on top of warm popcorn instead of butter to add the same creamy texture and extra flavor.

Ginger

Spicy, woody, and slightly tangy, this versatile root can be ground up, shaved, or candied. Although it's a great source of antioxidants, ginger has also been proven to alleviate nausea, arthritis, and migraines.

How I Enjoy It

Grate some fresh ginger over a fresh carrot salad, drop a cube of it into hot water with lemon for an invigorating infusion, or even add a bit to your cocktail for a spicy kick.

Mangoes

Perhaps my favorite midday snack, mangoes are low in calories and high in fiber, so they make you feel satiated longer. Since most cravings hit late in the day, try stashing a mango in your desk to quell your sweet tooth and deliver a powerful punch of vitamins. One small mango provides high doses of your recommended daily allowance for vitamin C, vitamin A, vitamin E, and fiber.

How I Enjoy Them

Add tropical flavor to boring salads by adding some juicy mango slices, or try swapping out tomatoes for mangoes to make a killer salsa you won't forget. And if you want the perfect complement to spicy foods, make an easy Indian lassi by combining equal parts of mango, yogurt, and milk in a blender with a teaspoon of honey and blend until smooth. Top it with a sprinkling of crushed pistachios, and you're in business!

Sweet Potatoes

Sweet potatoes are rich in vitamin A (the same betacarotene also found in carrots) and vitamin C, which are both powerful

antioxidants that remove free radicals, fight cancer, and can prevent skin problems associated with aging.

How I Enjoy Them

Forget fries! Slice sweet potatoes into wedges and top with
salt, pepper, and olive oil, and then bake at 350°F for 15–20 minutes, or until crispy, for a nutritious alternative to greasy potatoes. I also love slicing them in half and sprinkling them with a
mixture of brown sugar, cinnamon, and a dash of salt and then
baking them until tender for a sweet and savory side dish.

And Finally, the Yummiest Superfood Yet… Dark Chocolate

Yes, we all love sweets. But when it comes to chocolate, bitter
is better for the body. The benefits of chocolate come from
flavonols and antioxidants. Warning: only real cacao beans
contain flavonols, so look for chocolate that boasts a high per-
centage of cacao (60 percent or more). Or you could always
take a tropical vacay and travel to South America to grow some
chocolate firsthand! Dark chocolate also has fewer calories than
other varieties, and when eaten in moderation, it lowers unhealthy LDL cholesterol and prevents plaque from building up
in your arteries.

Aside from tasting good, chocolate stimulates endorphin
production, which releases a feeling of pleasure, and it contains
serotonin, which acts as an antidepressant (that explains the
chocolate craving during the breakup binge, not to mention the
menstrual cycle). And unlike salty chips, only one-third of the fat
in dark chocolate is bad for you.

You should look for pure dark chocolate or dark chocolate
with nuts (almond chocolates are scrumptious), orange peel, or

other flavorings. Avoid anything with caramel, nougat, or other fillings that counter the benefits of dark chocolate.

And last but not least (drumroll, please . . .), avoid the chocolate cow attraction! Research shows drinking milk with chocolate does not allow you to absorb the antioxidants found in chocolate. Besides, water quenches the sweetness better anyway.

How I Enjoy It

Every second I can! Dark chocolate stashed in my drawer during work, dark chocolate for Valentine's Day upon request, dark chocolate spread on toast. When I was a kid, I was allergic to cacao, but thank God I outgrew this allergy a few years ago. Now I'm home free and enjoying dark chocolate a few times a week.

There are things I don't recommend, like waxing your eyebrows, for example. I did that once and walked around with half an eyebrow missing. I spent two weeks filling in the big bare patch with dark brown eyeliner. Stealing your dad's razor to shave your bikini line is right up there too. You think he doesn't notice those long curly things that didn't wash out when you rinsed out his razor and put it back in its place? Superfoods, however, are on my recommended list. Not only do they keep me healthy, but they make me feel my best by providing me with strength, cancer fighting nutrients, and an extra little bounce in my step. I now call these superfoods my superpowers—my secret desire to be Superwoman has finally come true!

Shrimp 'n' Avocado

MAKES 4 SERVINGS

1 avocado, peeled, pitted,
    and cubed
2 ripe plum tomatoes
1 tablespoon chopped cilantro
1 shallot, chopped
1 pound cooked shrimp
Salt and pepper
2 tablespoons lime juice

Nutrition Facts

Amount Per Serving	
Calories 212	
Total Fat 8.7g	
Saturated Fat 1.4g	
Cholesterol 221mg	
Sodium 266mg	
Total Carbohydrates 8.8g	
Dietary Fiber 4.2g	
Sugars 3.2g	
Protein 25.6g	
Vitamin A 15%	Vitamin C 41%
Calcium 6%	Iron 23%

1. Stir together avocados, tomatoes, cilantro, shallots, and shrimp in a large bowl.

2. Season to taste with salt and pepper.

3. Stir in lime juice and serve cold.

Tip: Squeeze some lime over your avocado to prevent it from turning brown.

Chapter 7

If the Apron Fits, Wear It

As a CEO by Day and Chef by Night, I Really Get Down and Dirty in the Kitchen

I believe that each and every one of us is born with a special skill. My friend Kiki flirts with men and can practically swim in free cocktails. Stacy is a talented runner, while Alix can light up a room with her smile. Alexandra has a gift for languages and is fluent in five. Joanna and Mona are a gifted writers and I, well . . . I can cook. It was the best thing I ever learned. For me, cooking is both joyful and relaxing; it always warms the hearts of my loved ones. There is nothing like pleasing someone you care about by making them a special dish.

More important, cooking enables me to control my life. Unfortunately, because of my hectic, no-time-to-sleep schedule, cooking is not always an option. After much practice, however,

I've learned to find time for the simple, quick, and easy bases of cooking to ignite any appetite.

Working at Behind the Burner has been my best resource. Shooting videos with and interviewing chefs every day provides me with tips, tricks, and techniques I can use in my kitchen for life.

Many chefs have taught me how simple it is to coax brilliant flavors out of simple ingredients. And that's all it is, simplicity with a splash of technique. For example, Leah Cohen's pan-seared trout over roasted market vegetables for Behind the Burner was a quick run to a farmer's market and fish store, and about twenty minutes in my kitchen. The final product made it seem like I was attached to the stove all day. I also refer to the *Emeril 20-40-60: Fresh Food Fast* cookbook. This is a great tool to manage your time when cooking. You can select your recipe inspiration based on the amount of time you have—20 (think weeknight), 40 (think weekend), or 60 (think date with a guy who you want to take you to bed) minutes. This book avoids rushing and undercooked food, and has basically served as my crystal ball for the culinary world.

But let's rewind. Before the trout can get cooked, some shopping needs to be done. This is why you need to plan ahead. It's the Virgo in me that makes lists to shop for meals a few days in advance. Shopping for fresh, local, and organic produce is the only way to go. If you're like me, you'll make time on the weekends to food shop. On weeknights, I opt for making fish or a piece of chicken for dinner. I usually freeze fish in individual Ziploc bags so I can come home and make dinner for one or two. I'll marinate the fish in sesame oil or soy, let it sit for twenty minutes while I'm unwinding from work and then just broil or bake my fish and pair it with some steamed or lightly sautéed eggplant, spinach, or mushrooms. It's done in about five to ten minutes. The fish loads my system with a bunch of omega-3's—which I'm pretty sure you know all about by now. When it comes to chicken, I grill it and crust it with almonds, pecans, or even dried cranberries—all basic ingredients accessible at the local grocery store to make simple, flavorful, quality meals.

The key concept here is control—you can always control fat content by cooking at home and get the same flavor as you would at a restaurant. I hardly use oil, butter, or salt when cooking at home, something restaurant chefs always get away with. I buy lean meats and focus on whole grains. You'd be surprised if you ate my sweet potatoes, which don't have an ounce of cream. I also add color to my meals with fresh fruit, seasonal vegetables, or herbs, which deliver a mix of vitamins and nutrients.

Before you start cooking, always clean out the fridge and cupboard. If you have Fluff or Oreos up for grabs, it will completely defeat the hearty home-cooked meal you devoured for dinner. Limit sodium at home, not to mention any soda. Load up on brown sugar and other natural sweeteners that go perfectly with just about any fruit or squash. And get inventive! I usually freeze chicken stock and sauces (that take me hours to make on the weekend) in ice cube trays. This way, that labor lasts me weeks. When I need the sauce or stock, I pop out an ice cube's worth and use it. Brilliant, I know. Speaking of being efficient, I heat up red wine with tomato sauce, which can be used for fresh fish, seafood, meats, and pastas. Here, the sauce reinvents itself four different ways.

Cooking is fun alone but even better with company. My friends come over and get involved in the kitchen action. It's about the only exercise they get aside from chasing their toddlers and going to the gym. Nope, that sound is not our biological clocks ticking, it's the kitchen timer. Cooking is all pleasure. No epidural required.

Just keep in mind that you should cater to the needs of your company. One of my friends once brought a vegetarian date to my Cuban-themed dinner party. Clearly, she didn't have enough rice and beans (the only vegetarian option) because she ended up getting hammered on killer pineapple Bacardi Coco mojitos and spilling one all over my Indian silk rug. Lesson learned. Know your guest list before you spend time slaving over your guests. Their allergies and aversions will be the difference between an excellent and terrible meal.

Cooking not only allows you to control your fat calories, but also your portion sizes. As you know, at home you can save leftovers without feeling guilty about leaving food on your plate like you would at a restaurant. At my place there are always leftovers, which is why my neighbors love me. What I don't feed to them, I feed to my team the next day at work.

Too many people rely on frozen entrées for their weeknight dinners. You deserve better than chemicals heated up with radiation. If you are going to eat something out of the freezer, let it be last night's dinner that was homemade and that you decided to freeze for leftovers (just in case). A little cooking will take you a long way in the health department. If kitchen anxiety has got the best of you, just log on to www.behindtheburner.com and after watching a few episodes, your anxiety will melt away like butter. Your boyfriend will develop a newfound love for you and you'll be able to talk to your mom about something other than her hot flashes. Now, that makes us a site for sore eyes.

Finally, be creative. There is no RIGHT way to cook. After

all, this is not *Top Chef* and your guests are not weighing in on your skills at the judges' table. Look at recipes for ideas and inspiration. Treat them like a guide, not the gospel. Experimenting is the best way to learn. Believe me, aside from a broken soufflé, every kitchen disaster can be fixed. Stop looking. Get cooking.

411 on Homemade Juice

Fruits and veggies are obviously a very important part of our diets, but who has time to sit down and go through an entire bag of baby carrots? Not me. Which leads me to juicing: the quickest, easiest way to attain all the vitamins and minerals you want without having to eat five bell peppers in a row.

Here are the top three reasons to juice:

1. You can add a variety of fruits and veggies to your diet without having to eat them all individually. Become creative and mix your carrots and mangoes, or maybe even kiwis with bell peppers. Companies like V8 are doing it already. If you make your own, you can leave out any preservatives, high-fructose corn syrup, or sodium (and it's cheaper).

2. Juice is a simple way to consume lots of vitamins, minerals, and antioxidants in a single dose. Instead of scarfing down salads, you can get a concentrated dose of veggie nutrients by making them into juice.

3. Making juice is easy. You can make a lot of it and store it in the fridge for later, or you can mix it into various dishes or desserts. Make your own apple juice and add a little to our recipe, "Muffins That Won't Give You Muffin Top" (page

44); it will give the muffins just a smidge of tart flavor and since the juice is homemade, there's no extra sugar added.

Here's the best produce to use when juicing:

- Apples
- Oranges
- Mangoes
- Kiwis
- Carrots
- Grapefruit
- Strawberries
- Kumquats (great on their own, too!)
- Bell peppers
- Papayas
- Tomatoes
- Lemons
- Limes
- Spinach
- Wheatgrass
- Pears
- Celery

The sky is the limit! The best part about juicing is that you can make whatever you like. Try experimenting: for a really spicy take on an invigorating Bloody Mary, put a little turnip and spinach juice into the usual tomato/celery mixture with a splash of Worcestershire sauce and Tabasco. Fabulous, full of vitamins and minerals, and a great pick-me-up! Leave the vodka at the bar.

Flaky Fillets

MAKES 2 SERVINGS

2 (6-ounce) fillets red snapper
1 teaspoon freshly chopped garlic
Salt and pepper
¼ cup picante sauce
½ lime, juiced

Nutrition Facts

Amount Per Serving		
Calories 234.1		
Total Fat 2.9g		
Saturated Fat 0.6g		
Cholesterol 79.9mg		
Sodium 247.3mg		
Total Carbohydrates 3.6g		
Dietary Fiber 0.1g		
Sugars 2.6g		
Protein 44.9g		
Vitamin A 4.0%	•	Vitamin C 9.1%
Calcium 7.2%	•	Iron 2.4%

1. Preheat the oven to 350°. Line a baking sheet with a piece of aluminum foil and grease lightly.

2. Place the fillets on the foil and sprinkle with garlic and salt and pepper to taste. Spoon the picante sauce over the fillets and sprinkle the lime juice over the top. Bring the sides of the foil together and fold the seam to seal in the fish.

3. Bake for 7 to 10 minutes, or until the fish flakes easily with a fork.

Tip: To get the most juice out of your lime, make sure it is at room temperature before you cut into it.

Honey-Glazed Salmon

MAKES 4 SERVINGS

⅓ cup reduced-sodium soy sauce

¼ cup orange juice

¼ cup honey

2 green onions, thinly sliced

1 tablespoon olive oil

1 tablespoon sherry or apple
   juice

1 tablespoon minced fresh
   ginger root

1 pound salmon fillet

Nutrition Facts

Amount Per Serving	
Calories 324.9	

Total Fat 12.7g		
Saturated Fat 1.9g		
Cholesterol 80.5mg		
Sodium 784.7mg		
Total Carbohydrates 21.5g		
Dietary Fiber 0.3g		
Sugars 19.0g		
Protein 30.4g		

Vitamin A 2.7%	•	Vitamin C 2.6%
Calcium 2.6%	•	Iron 7.9%

1. In a large resealable plastic bag, combine the first seven ingredients. Add the salmon. Seal the bag and turn to coat; refrigerate for 1 hour, turning several times.

2. Line an 8-inch square baking dish with aluminum foil and grease it with nonstick cooking spray. Drain and discard the marinade. Place the salmon in the prepared pan. Bake at 350°F for 30 to 40 minutes, or until the fish flakes easily with a fork.

Tip: Salmon is loaded with omega-3 fats and promotes cardiovascular health.

Chapter 8

True Life

I'm Addicted to Sugar

Ever since Cocoa Krispies and Froot Loops were banned from me as a child, I realized the heartbreak I endured and silent treatment toward my parents were a result of nothing other than a severe sugar addiction. Fortunately, I took the candy route as opposed to the marijuana path some of my loser classmates followed in high school. Now, over twenty years later, I find myself undergoing withdrawal if my tongue doesn't encounter something sweet every few hours. Although I haven't broken my addiction, I have learned ways to better myself, aside from being a better baker (see Chapter 3, A Sweet Tooth for a Firm Ass). It's like the smoking patch for sugar-crazed people like me. Only the patch is more like a metaphor for a game plan in my wonderful world of reality Candy Land.

First, I began eating more natural sugars. As it was, I used to gag at the taste of the dreaded artificial sweeteners in the pink and blue packets, but every now and again I would indulge in Splenda. Coffee doesn't apply to me, but as for tea I've nixed my Splenda habit for good. Artificial sweeteners like this only succeed in helping you to crave more sugar: epic fail in my book. Studies have actually shown that artificial sweeteners do nothing more than mess with your brain, tricking it into thinking it is receiving calories and revving up the body's metabolism, which in turn just makes you hungrier.[1] I now use honey or raw sugar called turbinado. By eating natural sugars, you'll notice more things are sweeter than you realize, like bananas, mangos, cranberries, and anything with honey.

Throughout my years of culinary study, I've had an important revelation: refined, white sugar is disgusting. I know it isn't something most of you want to hear about these seemingly innocent white crystals, but they are bleached with sulfur dioxide, treated with phosphoric acid, and filtered with calcium hydroxide to remove the molasses, which is naturally present in sugar. Unfortunately, despite looking more "natural" because of its color, brown sugar is no better. It goes through the exact same process, but then they add molasses (which was just painstakingly removed) right back in.[2] Seem ass-backwards? It is. How did these confusing chemical compounds make their way into something as simple as sugar? I'm not going to rant about the science behind this, but I will say that switching to organic granulated sugar or turbinado is well worth it.

---

1 www.scientificamerican.com/article.cfm?id=artificial-sweetener-linked-weight-gain
2 www.thereluctanteater.com/2009/04/raw-sugar-vs-brown-sugar-vs-white-sugar

I'll also let you in on a sweet little secret of mine: agave. No, I'm not talking about tequila, although it is made from the same plant. Agave nectar is a mild, neutral-tasting, all-natural syrup that can be used in anything from sweetening drinks to baking. But there's something else about it that makes it a smarter sugar. Agave nectar has a low glycemic index, meaning that although it tastes sweet, it doesn't cause your blood sugar to spike when you eat it (unlike regular sugar, which does this and causes sugary cravings). Although it isn't calorie or carb free, it is 40 percent sweeter than granular sugars, so you can use less and get the same sweet results.

No high-fructose corn syrup. Because corn syrup is the cheapest sweetener, it is found as an ingredient in almost every prepackaged product. High fructose corn syrup is also found in soft drinks and even in some bread. The problem with this syrup is that it is heavily processed to extend the shelf life of products. In other words, you are willingly giving your body chemicals when eating products made with corn syrup. So how is one supposed to avoid this product that seems to creep its way into almost everything we eat? The easiest way is simply to avoid processed foods, which inevitably contain high amounts of corn syrup. That also goes for foods that contain added sugar, which usually comes in this form, so look for labels that read "No added sugar." This is especially true for beverages like juices and tea, so stop grabbing the first thing you see and start reading those labels!

No soda. Absolutely not. It's loaded with chemical flavorings, colorings, and corn syrup. I always argue that soda is just as bad for you as smoking. It rots your teeth, makes you put on weight, and has absolutely no nutritional value—the can label even says so, but not in so many words, I suppose. Soda's nickname is sugar. It's something that should never go in your mouth—and I don't care if "diet" is added to the label.

I also eat plenty of fiber. Soluble fiber stabilizes your blood sugar, which makes you feel full longer and have less cravings throughout the day. Soluble fiber is found in oatmeal, beans, fruits, and vegetables—a good replacement for the daily sugar dosage most can't overcome. Sure, fiber makes you shit. Better than making you inject yourself with insulin for diabetes, which sugar addictions may likely lead to.

Nutrition and medical facts aside, I think the most important rule for sugar is only to eat it when it's something you'll remember. Is that Snickers bar you scarfed down on the subway really going to stand out in your memory a month from now as a culinary triumph? Doubtful. Or the stale, store-bought birthday cake with crusty icing that your co-worker brought into the office? Hell, no. But that chocolate soufflé with vanilla crème anglaise from Le Cirque? Enjoy it now, and savor the memory until your next sugary splurge.

I'm not saying give up pastries and cookies and candy forever. I've already told you how you can make them lighter and healthier, but if you want to live long enough to see the next twenty, thirty years of fabulous fine dining to come, or rather, the birth of your grandchildren, to be more realistic, you'll break the addiction. If not, you're just as rotten as any low-life drug addict—with ugly teeth to prove it.

411 on Nutrition Bars

Nutrition bars can never be a substitute for the experience of sitting down to a "real" meal, but let's be honest, there are many instances where I am tied to my desk, stuck in a meeting, or simply don't have time for lunch. Rather than running to the vending machines or shoveling handfuls of popcorn down my throat, I grab a KIND Bar. Made from real ingredients (dried fruit and nuts) that you can actually see, KIND Bars are both delicious and satisfying. They come in a variety of flavor combinations and are tasty on their own or broken into pieces and mixed into plain Greek yogurt.

Supermarkets and gyms have entire isles dedicated to energy bars. Some are healthy, but many are loaded with as much sugar as a candy bar. Here are some guidelines to follow when choosing a bar:

1. Look at the label; you want a bar that is low in fat (anything more than 5 grams is pushing it) and without any trans fats.

2. High fiber bars will keep you satisfied; fiber is good for your heart and digestive tract.

3. Bars should have some protein to keep you feeling satiated. You should have about 1 gram of protein per kilogram of body weight each day. To figure out your weight in kilograms, simply divide your weight in pounds by 2.2.

4. Check the number of calories per serving (and check to make sure one bar is one serving!). Snack bars should have fewer than 200 calories, while a meal replacement bar might have as many as 400 calories. Keep the quantity below two teaspoons per serving.

5. Eat something "real" with the bar; I like a piece of fruit, yogurt, or carrot sticks.

Chapter 9

Beyond Metamucil

Why Hot Chicks Need Fiber

Ever wonder why your granny was always dumping a boatload of bran on her cereal in the morning? Or why your mom mixes up orange-colored powders? Here's a hint, ladies. They can't drop the kids off at the pool. Try to get that image out of your mind of your granny pushing so hard that she's turning blue in the face. Contrary to popular opinion, you don't have to stir orange powders into your water to get the daily amount of fiber you need and to stay regular.

Fiber, also known as roughage or bulk, is sugar and starch from plants. We need it to keep our system going. Fiber is essentially indigestible, so calories are not retained. Soluble fiber binds with water in our digestive tract and makes us feel full—it's good for weight loss and dieting. It slows glucose absorption, prevents blood sugar from spiking, prevents cravings, and the best part is, it curbs appetite. For those of you who eat way too much cheese, here's the good news: fiber can help lower cholesterol by absorbing fat from the food.

Now let's get down and dirty. Fiber promotes intestinal health and regularity (a.k.a. shitting). By cleansing the body regularly, fiber helps rid the body of toxins.

So, how much of this fun stuff do we need every day? The NFC recommends 25 to 32 grams per day. According to the Columbia University Institute of Human Nutrition, the average American barely consumes half of the recommended amount of fiber needed per day (10 to 15 grams). Now here's the story, you don't have to eat chewy, dry grains to get your fiber. Try fiber-rich fruits like figs, guava, raspberries, and apricots. Fiber-rich veggies include chick peas, artichokes, peas, and avocados. Go for these and you'll be shitting in no time.

Fruits
figs
guava
raspberries
apricots

Veggies
chickpeas
artichokes
peas
avocados

Herbal Tea
honey, cinnamon, lemon

Fact or Fiction?

You get as many vitamins and nutrients from fruit juice as you do from fruit.	*FICTION.* In the end, many fresh fruits contain more nutrients and fiber, because pasteurization of juices can destroy some vitamins and minerals.
A high-fiber diet helps prevent colon cancer.	*FACT.* Some studies show that a high-fiber diet will help prevent colon cancer.
Foods with soluble fiber cause less gas and bloating than those with insoluble fiber.	*FACT.* Soluble fiber dissolves in water. This type of fiber is found in oats, beans, peas, and citrus fruits. Insoluble fiber does not dissolve in water. When you take in insoluble fiber, it is digested by the intestines and interacts with the intestinal flora, thus causing gas and bloating.
Fiber can help control diabetes.	*FACT.* Fiber can assist in keeping your blood sugar levels even and can even cause reductions in blood sugar over time.

National Fiber Council: www.nationalfibercouncil.org

CHEAT
SHEET

Chapter 10

Serving Size Sexy

Training for the Portion Retarded

For any foreigners heading to America, I always think they should prepare themselves for one thing and one thing only: PORTIONS! Welcome to the land of supersize this and upgrade that where control seems to be missing from our vocabulary. Come on people, are you really hungry for two slices of pizza, two servings of pasta, and a 14 oz. steak every time you dine out? And I am sure you are not dying of hunger, or starving. Unless you've been in the desert for days surviving some sort of drought and famine, which I'm sure is a common occurrence for your everyday life. Please . . .

Well, instead of complaining about the enormous amount of shit we eat every day, I'm just not going to eat it all. The key word here is "all." To manage your weight, or hopefully, lose a little, you must watch how much food you eat during a sitting. Yes, you can have chocolate, but a piece, not the whole bar (a mistake you know you make). Yes, you can have pasta, but a cup, not a pile of it. Just think of each dish as your cheating ex-boyfriend with a bit of flavor. Instead of damage control, go with portion control.

The best way to figure out how much you need is by relating the amount that you consume to day to day objects you might see around your home (or in your gym bag). For example, a tennis ball's worth of broccoli can help you stay in the game by providing you with just the right amount of nutrients. A hockey puck sized bagel portion keeps you carb happy. Ready to slice that calorie intake in half? As they say, game, set, match!

The Food	The Amount	Equals . . .
Fish	3 oz.	A deck of cards
Meat/Poultry	3 oz.	A deck of cards
Tofu	3 oz.	A cassette tape
Beans	½ cup, cooked	A light bulb
Apple	1 cup/whole apple	A baseball
Dried Fruit	¼ cup	A golf ball
Orange Juice	1 cup	A tennis ball
Salad Greens	1 cup	A baseball
Baby Carrots	1 cup	A tennis ball
Baked Potato	1 small, plain	A computer mouse
Broccoli	1 cup	A tennis ball
Hummus	2 tbsp	A shot glass
Rice	½ cup	An ice cream scoop
Pancake	1 flapjack	A DVD
Pasta	1 cup	A tennis ball
Bagel	½ bagel	A hockey puck
Cheese	1½ oz.	4 stacked Monopoly dice
Ice Cream/Frozen Yogurt	1 cup	A tennis ball
Peanut Butter	2 tbsp	A shot glass
Extra Virgin Olive Oil	1 tsp	Tip of your thumb
Salad Dressing	2 tbsp	A shot glass

Chapter II

Takeout Tactics

Getting Tough When the Inevitable
To-Go Temptation Strikes

There are days where the thought of creating a meal for your-self is akin to that of curing AIDS or erecting the Great Wall of China. We've all experienced them. That cute guy I've been interested in decided he had better things to do for dinner (his loss) and my workload decides to double in size due to a late-running video shoot. Lean Cuisine is the last thing I want to reach for. Overly processed chemically enhanced food? No thank you! The kitchen is not at the top of my mind, even if it involves a thirty-minute Rachael Ray recipe. But with a quick pressing of buttons on my Crackberry, I can have my favorite meal in my apartment quickly and easily, without fuss. Life can get complicated and ordering in is a simple solution to slic-ing and dicing my way to a hurried meal. Despite being easy, it takes a bit of thought to order the proper meal to satisfy hunger and diet needs. Here are a few healthy takeout ordering tips that won't end in an extra Physique 57 class.

Veggie Love

While that heaping pile of chicken wings with the irresistible side of bleu cheese seems like a great idea in the starving moment, the calories you'll pack on from merely biting into it will cause your waist to expand like nobody's business. Only, it *will* be your business when it's time to shop for a size up on jeans that next month. No thank you. Instead, opt for more veggie-friendly choices, like a fresh garden salad (dressing on the side) or a side of steamed edamame. Lo mein can be just as tasty when the noodles are replaced with brown rice, especially when you request strictly veggie. Soba noodle soup is a winter favorite. Avoid high-calorie water chestnuts and baby corn; opt for extra bean sprouts or broccoli instead. No more feeling guilty for having little time to cook a five-course meal. Takeout no longer has to be the cause of little the white lies we tell our nutritionist. It can be just as good as anything made in a kitchen, if you choose wisely.

Forget the Fried, Savor the Steamed!

I know those fries topped with melted mozzarella are just bellissimo after a bad day (or night), but they hit you hard with an outrageous calorific punch. Buffalo wings and onion stems might as well be a train ride to two months on a health farm. Avoid extra time in the gym by ordering food steamed or grilled. Make sure to check condiment contents as well; if a food is steamed but smothered in a particular sauce, the whole purpose is negated. If you grab a burger, avoid the cheese and ask them to pile on the tomatoes and lettuce for a nutritional boost. When it comes to Chinese, think steamboat to China. Order steamed dumplings, steamed brown rice, steamed broccoli, steamed everything. If you must indulge in fattening sauces, ask for them on the side. If you do this often enough, they'll get the hint for future orders. Oh, and by the way, just because you order steamed vegetables for takeout, does not mean you "deserve" half a creamy cheesecake for dessert. Healthy takeout can be a great tactic if you follow through with it for the entire meal.

Saucy Is a Great Attitude, Not a Great Additive

Sure, a plate piled with chicken Alfredo seems like a delectable treat after a long day at the office, but the sauce is loaded down with butter and heavy cream. Barbecue chicken and extra sauce might as well be Siamese hips, attached at the bone, literally. Hot wings do not equal a hot bod. Many takeout foods are empty calories: heavy on the calories and light on filling you up. Ever wonder why four spare ribs and two fried-rice bowls later, you're still hungry? My point, exactly. But if you truly feel the need for sauce or dressing, order it on the side. With salads, anything vinaigrette will be to your benefit. Balsamic is the usual go-to for me. Check for low-fat or no-fat options at the salad bar and in the grocery store. Better yet, make the dressing yourself. It's supereasy and you can control the oil. Replace oil with fresh orange or pomegranate juice for the most flavorful dressing you've ever had.

Smaller Portions

The local Chinese takeout doesn't just come with an entrée. Saving some of that extra rice for later makes the next day's dinner easy to throw together, especially if you're running late due to a snafu at work or a delayed train—I've experienced both on numerous occasions. Many Italian places give at least three portions for one person; let your eyes be bigger than your stomach. Ordering in with friends allows sharing, which will prevent you from overstuffing your face with chicken parm and penne à la pound-packer . . . or vodka, same dish. It also lowers the probability of staining your clothes. The fewer portions I have, the less likely I am to spill sauce on my shirt. I still manage to get it all over my face, but that's another story.

Don't Touch That Coke

Avoid soda pop at all costs! Give it up like you gave up keg stands after college. Okay, maybe it took you a few years to give up those keg stands?! A syrupy, sugar-loaded beverage may seem the easiest route to go, but water is truly your friend when ordering out. Water is free at home. Don't buy into that 2-Liter Coke special from Pizza Hut or Domino's—I even hear some Chinese places are doing it too, depending on your order. It's a deadly trap. Being a food slut is perfectly acceptable, but who wants to be a Coke whore? Water also helps fill you up, so going overboard with entrées is less likely. Even if you're craving that Diet Coke, step back. Just like all the fried crap no-no's we spoke about, Coke's refined, fake sugars will come back to bite you in the butt! I mean, who wants an ass that could swallow up a thong, anyway? Certainly not me.

Now, if you find yourself really craving that extra flavor, add some lemons to ice water or even order an unsweetened ice tea. Be careful about putting Splenda or Sweet'N Low into drinks. These sweeteners can do more harm than good, despite being low calorie. In the winter months, ordering green tea from a Japanese restaurant is a bonus over hazelnut coffee from Dunkin' Donuts or a Starbucks skinny vanilla latte. The only thing skinny about that latte is the coffee sleeve preventing your chubby hand from burning. I know most "flavored" coffees are sugar free, but not after you request a light and sweet beverage to go. There is nothing sweet about Sweet 'n Low, and there is definitely nothing splendid about Splenda. Unless you consider cancer in the near future and wide hips a pleasant surprise, Herbal tea is the way to go. Plus, now you can "go green" in more ways than just recycling.

Never Be Afraid to Ask

Failing to ask what's going into your food is like forgetting to read a business contract before you sign it—DUMB! The food you consume can cause permanent and constant damage to your body that may be irreversible. In New York, restaurants are supposed to report the calorie content of their food; if it's not visible, ask. Nothing bad ever came from asking questions, especially because it is important to know what you're eating. That veggie burger may seem like a good idea, but what tops it may be surprising. Same goes for that California grilled chicken salad. They leave out what's so Californian—or should I say caloric—about the "healthy side." Ordering healthy with the eyes doesn't always translate to your stomach or your body. Knowledge is power!

Eating is like sex. When you eat, you should take full pleasure in the action, disregarding anything else in the world for that moment. Never eat in front of the TV. This also means don't eat while stalking Facebook walls or Twittering your brains out, popping a spoonful of cereal in your mouth every other tweet—

doing this will cause you to overeat. You will be too distracted to realize that you are full, and worst of all, you won't even remember how good the meal was because you're so goddamned focused on social media rather than using meal time to be social with people that aren't on a screen. Eat slowly at the table and savor every single bite of your meal without interruptions. About 25 percent of Americans eat too fast. Avoid traveling while eating too. I can never understand how anyone thinks it's healthy to walk while you eat. Not only do you look like a heifer stuffing a carb-infested bagel with way too much cream cheese in your mouth, but your body can't digest well on the move. And no, walking while eating does not equal "working off your food." Eating is a human necessity. We deserve to enjoy what we put in our mouths. Being fully immersed in a meal is the only way to do so.

Ordering in is supposed to be a relaxing experience, no whining about dirty dishes—that's what they invented recycled paper plates for! Be aware of the food you consume; strive for slow and conscious eating to fill you up as you chew. The kitchen will remain spotless, the body full, and the stomach completely satiated. With dinner out of the way, I can luxuriate in my spotless home and pack extra meals in my fridge for later. After my amazing meal in, I have extra time to get ready for my night out.

Chapter 12

Ethnic Eats

When Culture Invades My Stomach . . .
Watch Out!

When it comes to food, I consider myself to be hungry for: Italian, Mexican, German, Indian, Greek, Spanish, French, Japanese, Irish, and pretty much for food from anywhere else on the globe. I eat everything these countries have to offer, from fettuccine Alfredo to chorizos to churros con chocolate. Fortunately, I've learned that if I eat the entire cuisine every country has to offer, I'll most likely become the size of that country. Now when dining out, I stick to six main options from around the world that won't make my stomach the size of the globe.

Mexican

Hola! We all know guacamole is a must, but when dining Mex, try not to eat the whole basket of chips that accompany it.

Remember, although avocados are great for cleaning the arteries, they are rich in fat. Have two to three chips and be done.

Next, try to stick to the fish selections. Bye-bye beef tacos and cheesy enchiladas. One enchilada can have over 200 calories. That's 600 calories if you have three! And trust me, one will not fill you up. Instead, go for shrimp or fish Veracruzana or salmon served with tomatoes, greens, and Mexican seasoning. For you fish haters, cook tacos at home and purchase lean beef and veggies without the rice and beans. Rice and beans are just a pile of carb mush that will make you become best friends with the toilet. No action for you that night, trust me—just stay clear. Have I mentioned the gas that goes along with beans? You get my drift. Most Mexican restaurants offer salads and tortilla soups. Stick to those choices. And if you must get dessert, share it. However, I'd prefer one margarita over flan anytime. You must pick and choose your food battles, especially with this calorie-laden cuisine.

Italian

Ciao! If you want to consider yourself a bella, the creamy sauces and family-style pasta dishes must go a-walking. Sorry to be harsh, but Italian dining is a nightmare in progress for the body. Yes, I sometimes dream of the moist garlic bread, penne alla vodka, pizza, chicken Parmesan (which is far from a true Italian dish anyway); how could one resist?! I know soup is not exactly your idea of a kick-ass Italian meal, but minestrone soup is rather tasty and won't give you pasta thunder thighs, as I like to call them. Lentil soup is also a personal favorite of mine. When cooking or ordering pasta, always order whole wheat—it tastes exactly the same as regular pasta. Avoid the Alfredo and vodka sauces and extra sprinkles of grated Parmesan cheese unless you want to taste what is not-so-great for your waist. Rather, to stay in shape and still enjoy the food, just stick to simple tomato-based sauces and you can't go wrong. Add steamed vegetables to your entrée instead of the extra helping of bread for dipping. I'm sure you've had bread and sauce enough times in your life that you can resist from now on. And the cheesecake—forget about it. Unless of course you're planning on having that as your meal, and nothing else. Not a good idea! Personally, I prefer to enjoy some whole wheat pasta, chicken, and salad rather than a lump of cake fat on my dish (unless it's chocolate of course . . . kidding). For pizza, stick to thin crust without the pepperoni pound-packing crap. If anything, get mushrooms or even salad pizza. Most restaurants offer whole wheat crust too, so take advantage. Italian dining does not have to equal preparation for weight gain every time you dine out. And don't wear leggings or stretch pants when eating this cuisine as an easy escape. You can mangia! As long as you stick to your limit. Trying every flavor of gelato or a whole bowl of tiramisù in one sitting is just unacceptable. You want to fit into that sexy Italian leather bustier, don't you?

German

I am not quite sure if it's possible to eat healthy German food—unless your diet is strictly beer and sausage, which is just sad. But if you must, I'd enjoy some bratwurst braised with apples, cabbage, and carrots. Usually bratwurst is marinated in beer, so I would avoid eating any bread with the sausage. If you choose to have schnitzel, go easy on it. A few bites is enough. Stay away from German potato salad. You're better off having a baked potato with some sauerkraut and low-fat sour cream. Instead of eating German spaetzle—or rather, noodles smothered in egg yolk—opt for trout, a popular fish in this cuisine. Asparagus is a common side dish and is nutritious, best served sautéed with garlic—do not fry and bread the asparagus and think you are still eating healthy! If you must eat bread, German breads are in fact far better than Italian heroes and America's dreadful white loaves. Try German rye wheat or pumpernickel bread—it allows healthy and bread to actually coexist.

Japanese

Ever since America decided sushi dates beat out coffee dates, Japanese cuisine has thrived. However, sushi itself can be a killer. But let's backtrack. When eating Japanese food, do not order any fried shrimp or tempura. Imagine sticking a whole piece of broccoli in a deep fryer—you are simply demeaning the value of veggies; it's pure evil. Instead, edamame, which are delicious soybeans, make a good choice for the appetizer. You can suck on a million prior to your entrée without feeling bloated. Stay away from spicy tuna rolls and Philadelphia cream cheese avocado rolls. Clearly, if cream cheese is not healthy on a bagel, why would it be healthy in a roll of rice? Avoid any eel selections, as they tend to be fatty. Rather, have sushi as you would in healthy Japan, not supersized America. Order sashimi, which is sliced fish à la carte that omits the rice. Veggie rolls and anything with salmon are also a plus. Also, try to request brown rice instead of white for your sushi rolls. The extra charge is better than the extra pound. And, of course, low-sodium soy sauce on everything, if you want your Louboutins to fit on the way out of Nobu!

Irish

Most people think of three things when it comes to Irish cuisine: corned beef, cabbage, and soda bread—stupid, stupid, stupid. St. Patrick's Day is not the only day to have Irish food. Take advantage of Irish stews, usually made from lots of wheat and barley. If you have a choice, choose lamb for the meat. Fortunately, Irish meats are served with boiled root veggies, such as potatoes, carrots, turnips, and parsnips. Steer clear of bacon and sausage breakfasts; instead, enjoy the heartiness of meat broth and the veggies this country has to offer.

Indian

From rich, creamy curries to grated coconut with curry leaves, there is plenty of temptation when dining out on Indian cuisine. Portion control is the mantra here, guys. Don't continue eating because your remaining cauliflower needs another naan. A good choice for a healthy breakfast is a sprouted mung salad over roti. Spritz on some lemon juice and savor the fabulous dance on your tongue. If leaning toward an Indian buffet, beware! Idlis, or steamed fermented rice cakes, served with a lentil soup like sambhar is also a good choice. Stay away from deep-fried vadas and uttapams. Those are for the farmers doing manual labor all day. If you must have some crunch, ask for a roasted pappadum. Roasted is the key.

Mainstream choices for healthy meals are plentiful. All varieties of vegetables, daals (lentil-souplike dish), roasted meats, and grilled fish make delicious no-guilt options with whole wheat bread (rotis). Steer clear of the parathas—superdelicious but superfatty. Most Indian food is eaten with raita, yogurt with cucumbers. It is a must to cool off the heat from the spices, unless you like a permanent fire in your mouth.

Desserts are normally prepared seasonally. Homemade would be the way to go. My grandma makes her own gajjar ka halwa by simply boiling carrots in milk and dressing with a sprinkle of sugar and blanched almonds. This beats the storebought version made with cream and tons of butter. When craving sweets in the summer, a low-fat option is ragsullas, steamed ricotta balls in a sugary syrup. They are divine, with a mouthwatering simple goodness that melts away in your mouth.

Chapter 13

The Four O'Clock Problem

Snacking Smart

My dad jokes that "snacker" is the title of my mom's occupation, aside, of course, from yoga queen, spiritual preacher, health nut, and Internet junkie. He mocks her for eating about a million dollars worth of fruit a year, giving her a look every time he walks into the kitchen. Well, like mother like daughter. I think he should have changed my middle name to "grazer" on my birth certificate, leaving me justified for my snacking fixation.

While writing most of this book, including this chapter, I decided there was no better inspiration than placing my Mac on the kitchen table. What better inspiration than a room full of food? Despite the motivation from the aroma of vegetables roasting and shiny fruit sitting in a basket, the kitchen gave me easy 24/7 access to snacks. The trick is not to stop snacking, but to make healthy choices. In fact, the more you snack, the faster your metabolism and the less hungry you are throughout the day.

Shop Smart

By now, you know I'm always flying through New York City like I'm racing toward some finish line in a 10k marathon. Aside from my happy foods, most of the time I need accessible snacks to get me through the long day. I do this by stocking up on everything from fruit, veggies, nuts, and occasionally 100-calorie packs you can buy in bulk at a local Target (if I'm feeling particularly desperate and willing to eat chemicals); however, don't be that person who eats five 100-calorie packs as his or her meal. Sorry to break it to ya, but you just ate your lunch and dinner in bite-size flattened Oreos or Wheat Thins.

I'm all about fruits and veggies—I could have written a Barney song better than "Apples and Bananas" if they'd asked me. Contrary to the illogical, expensive Atkins diet or fad fitness manuals—you people didn't fool me—fruit actually has tons of antioxidants. I'm always peeling an orange or eating a pear, rather than portioning out the limited range of fruits I am "allowed" to eat.

Eating fruit alone is the best way to do it. Fresh fruit provides for better digestion and is way better than the "wannabe" fruit. You can even freeze fruits like cherries or grapes, which allow you to suck on the fruit longer, sort of like a flavored ice cube. I do, however, prefer applesauce to apples, which is both filling and healthy, simply because it's just a puree of cooked apples. I like regular apples from time to time too. Mushy Royal Galas are my favorites. You can usually find me on the public bus snacking on red apples. I don't like the tart Granny Smith ones; those I save for my best friend, Stacy. They also hold up well while baking. I pair my apples with almond butter that somehow always ends up stuck in my hair. This happens, oh, about every other week. It's almost as bad as chewing gum, but that's a whole other issue. Almond butter is also a great source of protein. You can even throw a bunch of fresh berries like blackberries and raspberries in a blender with some low-fat frozen yogurt, pour it in a Thermos, and you have a drink to keep you full most of the day. Fruit smoothies sure beat out any $5.00 Starbucks that goes cold after about five minutes.

Now for the veggies. These are easy because they require one trip to the grocery store and a few Ziploc bags. Just load up on carrots, celery, broccoli, red peppers, or any other veggies you prefer. Take fifteen minutes to place them in Ziploc bags and throw them in the fridge. In the morning, all you have to do is jump in the fridge, grab them, and go. You can eat a pound of veggies and not gain a centimeter on your waist. Now that's empowering. Get creative. Hummus, rather than thigh-thickening ranch dressing, goes well with carrots. Celery sticks are also great with almond butter. Stick to the natural stuff. Processed foods are made only to be paired with a neon lunchbox.

Five Best Protein-Packed Snacks

1. *Cottage cheese:* This old-school staple may seem boring, but cottage cheese is a versatile and healthy midday snack that won't leave you craving a Snickers. Sweeten it up with fresh fruit and a drizzle of honey, or go savory with sliced veggies and a sprinkling of sea salt for a protein-packed afternoon treat.

2. *Almond butter:* Everyone knows almonds are good for you, but what they don't know is that portion control is crucial. Polishing off an 8-oz. bag of almonds can set you back as much as 800 calories; instead, opt for a couple tablespoons of almond butter spread on whole- wheat toast.

3. *Dry-roasted edamame:* Steamed edamame isn't exactly a purse-friendly snack, so I opt for the dry-roasted variety. These green beans pack up to 15 grams of protein in just a quarter of a cup, but make sure to choose the lightly-salted version.

4. *String cheese and whole-wheat crackers:* String cheese is cheap, portable, and a sure-fire way to prevent overeating. I pack one stick along with a few whole-wheat crackers for an easy afternoon snack.

5. *Greek yogurt:* I started eating Greek yogurt years ago and haven't looked back since. Not only is this my breakfast staple, but I also use it to add nutrition to smoothies for a per- fect post-workout drink.

Snack Wisely

Now, once you have these snacks, use them wisely at work. I'm teaching both myself and you that your desk drawer does not need to be renamed the chocolate chest. Unless your office is smack in the middle of Dylan's Candy Bar. I came to my senses on this issue recently when Behind the Burner received a lovely package of endless Scharffen Berger chocolate bars. I'd break off a piece every few hours, and by the end of week one I realized half the bars were somehow missing—wondering who the culprit was?

If you stock your office solely with Post-its, pens, thumbtacks, paper clips, and the occasional stack of cookbooks on the windowsill, not to mention the messy piles of shoes blocking the doorway, food will not be an issue. Get your ass up and walk to the kitchen—already two minutes of exercise for the day! That's progress. And always keep water in your kitchen fridge, both at home and at work. If you're one of those Diet Coke fanatics or Propel people, get over it! Just add a little bit of honey or cinnamon, or even lemon, and you have flavor. I also do the whole herb and spices thing to my food. Roasted squash with cinnamon or grapefruit with a little brown sugar adds some spark into your mission for healthy eating. I also bring some cheeses to the office. I'm a fan of Babybel, even the Babybel cheese spread, which is awesome paired with multigrain toast or whole-grain crackers. I even prefer the spread to butter on a multigrain English muffin. Tuna without mayo is also great on whole-grain crackers. I tend to mix it with some celery and scallions as a midmorning bite. PMS'd? Try tuna with hot sauce, cucumbers, and onion—works miracles around that time of the month.

I will admit some snack habits are still in the works. I always opt for fresh produce, but I pick a few processed/packaged items (try not to go for ones loaded with sugar and sodium) for when I'm on the go (they last a lot longer, especially when you are traveling). Jell-O pudding, the fat-free kind, is one such treat. They are a bit high on the sweet side of things, but I enjoy them . . . especially the chocolate ones.

Pickles are also a great snack. I learned this from speaking with health expert Dr. Stephen Gullo on one of our shoots from Behind the Burner. He also told me about Ricola gumdrops that are zero calories and full of lemony flavors. If you have some sort of oral fixation where you must eat even though you know you're not starving, buy these with pocket change.

Listen up, snack heads. The point is not just to snack mindlessly like some famine is about to take over America. Chain eating is just as bad as chain smoking in my book. It doesn't allow your body to digest properly and you'll never be able to tell when you're fully satisfied. Only snack if you're really hungry. Eat, wait a little bit, and then eat another snack if you are still hungry!

Smart Snacking

If you are craving . . .	Eat . . .	Because . . .
Carbs	French Meadow Bakery Bagels	Eat the sprouted 16-grain & seed bagels made from a blend of sprouted grains and legumes and packed with crunchy flax seed and sunflower seeds. Each all-natural bagel provides 14 grams of protein and 10 grams of fiber. These bagels are organic, yeast free, and gluten free.

If you are craving . . .	Eat . . .	Because . . .
Something healthy on the go	KIND bars	KIND bars are all-natural fruit and nut bars made from ingredients you can see and pronounce. They are filled with protein. My favorite is the KIND almond & apricot. It's delicious, all natural, gluten free, wheat and dairy free. It's a rich source of fiber and low in sodium.
Something salty	Food Should Taste Good Multigrain Chips	If you are about to reach for potato chips . . . DON'T. Food Should Taste Good has a healthier alternative with flax, sunflower and sesame seeds, and loads of flavor.
Something sweet	Driscoll berries and a little clover honey	Berries are a great source of vitamins, minerals, fiber, and phytochemicals. A cup of berries has less than 100 calories. Honey is a natural sweetener without chemicals.

Cinnamon Sugar Applesauce

4 apples, peeled, cored,
    and chopped
¾ cup water
¼ cup brown sugar
1 teaspoon ground cinnamon

Nutrition Facts

Amount Per Serving

Calories 134.7

Total Fat 0.5g
  Saturated Fat 0.1g
  Trans Fat 0.0g
Cholesterol 0.0mg
Sodium 5.6mg
Total Carbohydrates 39.8g
  Dietary Fiber 4.0g
  Sugars 18.3g
Protein 0.3g

Vitamin A 1.5%	•	Vitamin C 13.4%
Calcium 3.0%	•	Iron 4.0%

1. In a saucepan, combine the apples, water, sugar, and cinnamon. Cover and cook over medium heat for 15 to 20 minutes, or until the apples are soft.

2. Allow to cool, then mash with a fork or potato masher.

Tip: An apple kept at room temperature becomes softer ten times faster than if refrigerated.

Chapter 14

Room Service

Dining Secrets from a Frequent Flyer

If I could have one superpower, flying would be off my list, mainly because I do it all the time. I practically travel for a living and not just to keep my American Airlines platinum status. We've filmed in Boston, Los Angeles, San Francisco, Dallas, several cities in Spain, and the list goes on and on. When it comes to cross-country jet-setting, I always keep my tummy in check. I start every flight with a note to self: stuff snacks in my carry-on. That's because I'm all about the carry-on. I could travel for two weeks with just my carry-on and be fine. My clothes fold up to the size of thin notebooks. It's always a fun time when airport security realizes I have more snacks than shoes in my Tumi rollerboard.

When traveling, always remember two things: A: resist temptation; B: be prepared.

Taking Flight

For long flights, I always bring Ziploc bags with me full of almonds, flax seed, dried fruit (particularly apricots, cranberries, and dried cherries), sunflower seeds, and anything else that goes nicely with the word "healthy." You don't want to be eating all the garbage airlines usually hand out. And you sure as hell don't want to be the person eating six bags of peanuts on a plane.

Now, when flying any airline you must avoid the meat option. The quality of meat served on airplanes is scary, especially when the temperature ranges from overcooked to rock-solid stone cold. It'll usually have your stomach doing a 360—believe me, there's enough turbulence on most planes, we don't need any turbulence in the tummy. Vomiting on planes equals puke smell for the remainder of the flight. There's no pulling over to the closest cloud station—and most people think getting carsick is bad. Just avoid the meat. In fact, if you are a frequent flyer, most airlines allow you to call in advance to request a meal. Always request the vegetarian option, and sometimes there is even a low-fat category, mainly if you fly first class. Aside from the hot towels and comfy seats, you'd think first class on American Airlines had their own private bakery. My weakness is their chewy chocolate chip cookies and sometimes their brownie sundaes. I struggle against myself for resistance and look like the idiot staring at her food tray while mumbling against the temptation. I almost always give in. I try to salvage my poor decision by ordering skim milk with my cookies.

If you don't fly first class, don't fret. Lucky for you, cookies won't be an issue. You can also bring some apples and a pound of toasted pumpkin seeds, or some whole-grain cereal along for snacking. And don't forget water. For flights two to seven hours long, bring a 16-ounce bottle, and ask the flight attendant for some lemon if you want flavor. For flights to Europe or Asia, bring two bottles. This way you can keep yourself full by chugging water most of the trip and eventually passing out to your iPod. However, avoid drinking a lot of water if you find yourself in one of those long middle-row seats—getting up to use the bathroom in a box toilet is never pleasant—unless of course you enjoy annoying people. Either way, avoid the narrow variety of Sprite, Coke, and Diet Coke drinks that don't even come with caps. It's like they expect you to down a whole can of soda as if it's Gatorade after a marathon. Just stick to your own sugar-free, ulcer-avoiding, non-bone-depleting water beverage, please.

One thing I can always control on a plane is the booze. I don't even know why alcohol is still an option on flights. They might as well offer you free Xanax pill-popping privileges if they want passengers to pass out. Alcohol does not make you relax. In fact, it sometimes causes people more anxiety on a plane. In addition, it dries out your skin. As it is, I have to gob on a load of Vaseline under my eyes so they don't dry out from the stale plane air. One time my friend (who shall remain nameless) thought it'd be cute to attend Margaritaville in the airport when our plane was delayed on the way back from a tropical vacation. Let's just say she was hugging the porcelain (or shall I say plastic?) bowl for the duration of the flight.

Road Tripping

If you're traveling by car, lucky you. You can avoid going through security and having them assume your lip gloss is some sort of secret weapon. But more important, you can pack entire meals in your car. Stock up on fresh vegetables and sandwiches on whole wheat, stored in coolers—I'd avoid any form of mayo if I were you. Turkey and tuna wraps fit easily in Ziploc bags. You can cut the wraps into bite-size pinwheels to make them easier to pop in your mouth. Bring boxes of whole wheat crackers, packs of water, and of course, a must-have variety of nuts. Trail mix with dried fruit and granola is also great to bring on road trips, but avoid the mixes with the M&M's—it defeats the whole point of eating nature's food. Fill up Tupperware with cubed fruit. When stopping at rest stops, look for single-serving whole-grain cereals or protein bars (if you must ingest chemicals). But watch out, many protein bars are high in calories, so you may be better off with some low-fat yogurt. Only choose a hot breakfast sandwich if your only other option is a donut or muffin. But I'm not talking sausage, egg, and cheese McMuffin sandwich here. You might as well buy the donut and the muffin to equal the 450 calories this sandwich contains.

I sometimes drive the Behind the Burner crew when we have shoots in Boston or Connecticut. Although they think my driving is a hazard to American civilians, they always thank me for the healthy snacks in my car and also for never stopping at a rest stop with a Starbucks or a Burger King. If you stop there, you might as well eat what they have to offer, so what's the point if you know the stuff's bad for you? This goes for airports as well. Avoid any calorie-filled drinks at Starbucks! I don't care if they're giving out free eggnog frappucinos or caramel lattes. It's all poison to me. If you go to Starbucks, get their fruit and cheese platter. Same goes for McDonald's: ask for the fruit and walnut salad. Anything is better than sugar-saturated whipped coffees. This is also not the time to be opening a greasy bag of salt and vinegar chips. Think road to thin heaven, not road to heart attack hell.

Checking In

The hotel is a whole other story. You'd think when I stay at the Mohegan Sun to do a shoot at Todd English's Tuscany, along with more food from none other than Jasper White, they'd realize I have enough food to entertain myself with all weekend. Nope! Same goes for the Ritz in San Francisco. There was a chocolate basket in the room full of enough chocolate-covered strawberries and candies to feed all the hotel guests on my floor. I was particularly touched by the Behind the Burner logo that was made out of chocolate. The thought was quite nice, but served as a temptation all week. I'll admit I recently chased a housekeeper from the Ritz in Miami down the hallway to get a few more dark chocolates that were placed on my bed. Two were not enough! So, please just imagine what this chocolate basket put me through. But what I do is save these gourmet treats for my friends. They get more excited when I leave on trips now because they know I'll bring home some massive edible chocolate sculpture fit for any girl's wine night.

I've also become a pro at tackling the room service menu. I order salads with dressing on the side and lean proteins; I always request my vegetables steamed, and ask for heavy sauces on the side. I try to keep a food budget every day. I have a small budget for my unhealthy foods, like the chocolate-covered strawberries or the days when I want a little cream sauce on my chicken.

Room service is a piece of cake when it comes to the continental nightmare of a breakfast. Try to stick to egg white omelets with veggies. These people are chefs that are paid to serve you, so do not be afraid to ask. You do not want a fried egg splattered on a thick New York bagel just before you're about to be filmed. Berries and yogurt are also a plus. Avoid all the croissants and any type of Danish pastry.

Sometimes I carry cups of Greek yogurt with me if I'm not traveling too far. But always make sure you have a mini-bar to keep it cold (and not one of those weight-sensitive ones that charge you every time you move something around). If not, you'll either be stuffing your sink with ice to serve as the new fridge or chucking the yogurt good-bye. Oatmeal is also ideal for those little front pouches of your carry-on suitcase. Just add hot water when you get to the hotel, and some blueberries or bananas, and you have a hearty breakfast. My little secret is letting a piece of dark chocolate left on your pillow melt into your morning oatmeal the next day. It blows Cocoa Krispies out of the water, and it's healthier!

You don't need to use the hotel gym to stay in shape. I take a jump rope with me for the mornings—a hot pink jump rope, to be exact! It always makes for good conversation with the hotel maids. I also do some jumping jacks and crunches on the floor before starting my day. Just because you're on vacation doesn't mean your body goes dormant. And just because your company is paying for all the expenses on your trip doesn't mean you need to order everything on the menu. Try to eat like a normal human being. You can enjoy fruit and cheese platters. Just because you're on a business trip doesn't mean you have to go food crazy. And even for vacations, there is no need to splurge every night. You want to look and feel good during your getaway time, right?

Finally, pass on the minibar. Even if it's free, it doesn't mean you have to fuel up your liver. Save the booze for a night out with your friends, not a night in alone in a hotel room . . . that's lame.

Checking Out

At the start of my many culinary journeys, I used to eat like there was no tomorrow. But I soon realized there is a tomorrow, and I want to be around to see it in the most fit and fabulous way.

Chapter 15

The Morning After

Avoiding the Post-Thanksgiving/ Holiday Slump

Thanksgiving is my single favorite day of the year. Who needs Valentine's Day chocolates when you can have roasted turkey, smooth gravy, yams, and pumpkin pie? I'd probably have the chocolates in addition to all that too. No matter how good you are the week before, it is pretty possible that you will ignore all sense of reason on Thanksgiving Day. And then comes the weekend: leftovers of turkey soup, turkey sandwiches, and cranberry sauce with chestnut stuffing for a snack.

My mom doesn't like to waste, so we end up stuffing our faces with stuffing, and much more, all weekend. Now, instead of jiggling, my thighs begin gobbling. Once you're off the bandwagon it's easy just to give up. But DON'T . . .

Here's How I Cope on the Monday After . . .

Don't feel bad. Most of us feel guilty for everything we ate on turkey day and all the DVDs we watched while our families were playing football outside. So, you caught up on all the movies you hadn't seen in six months in one weekend. Oh and you ate nonstop snacks through each movie the entire weekend. Do not despair. What's done is done. Don't cry over spilled milk. Instead, let go of your guilt and start fresh.

Step Far, Far Away from the Scale

Do *not* weigh yourself, unless you want to feel completely and utterly hopeless from the few pounds that may show up the morning after hard-core turkey consumption. This is why I don't own a scale, but I know my friends get manic about jumping on it, constantly obsessing over one-pound movements in their weight. I think you should judge your health by how you feel (inside and out), not based on a number on a scale. Face it, you like to eat, you're a food slut and food sluts aren't anorexic. Think about how your clothes feel and how you look in them and don't sweat the digital digits. Most doctors are more concerned about how you look and feel rather than a dumb number on a metal square. If you regularly weigh yourself, just give yourself a break for a few days after your eating paradise weekend. All of those high-sodium Thanksgiving Day foods have you retaining water and you don't want to know how much. Just give yourself a few days to shed the water weight and then you can get back on the scale (if you have to).

Log It

Start your food log again. You will feel ashamed when you have to write down that you had two desserts in one sitting, or three, not to mention the quick scarfing down of your aunt's home-baked cookies that you forgot to count. You can even go to the dollar store and get a cheap, pretty notebook to record your daily eats.

Get Rid of the Garbage

Donate, regift, or throw out all the tempting foods from Thanksgiving. You already ate your dose, so let go of the rest.

Hit the Grocery Store

Stock up on fresh fruits, veggies, lean proteins, low-fat cheese, yogurt, and all of my favorite superfoods (see Chapter 6, Super-size It).

Channel Your Inner Chef

Cooking not only saves you money, but it saves you a few pounds. Most takeout foods, even the side of veggies you order just to feel good about yourself, come soaked in oil. Cooking gives you the control, and it's fun too! I tend to grill chicken and sauté veggies in garlic, and put them in my pasta, sprinkled with a little bit of Parmesan cheese. Oh and for those who think brown pasta is "just not the same," try the whole wheat pasta that is now white. I'm telling you, it's all a mind game you play with yourself. Not only is whole wheat pasta better for you, it also tastes the same as the regular kind. Cooking allows you to unleash your creative side and experiment with meals, especially when hosting dinner parties. Plus who wants to dig through the bottom of their overstuffed YSL downtown handbag to find singles to tip the Domino's delivery guy?

Bring the Bacon to Work

Bringing your own lunch keeps your wallet full. More important, it allows you to limit what you eat. Tired of the same daily routine: leave the office around noon, stop for a slice of pizza or a "healthy salad" drenched in ranch, then on your way back realize you just need that Starbucks Caramel Frappucino with whipped cream because lunch just wasn't enough? Ha, it's always the same. We want what we see and smell. Ever just want popcorn in the movie theater because you smell that buttery luscious snack everywhere you go, even though you just ate a big dinner minutes ago? Exactly. Instead, carry your lunch to work (it'll make for some good arm lifting). Tuna, homemade garden salads, cucumber sandwiches with chutney, chicken breast in a light sauce, and dinner leftovers are tasty options. If your office has a refrigerator, bring some balsamic dressing for the week. Bring a box of mesclun greens, a few fruits and nuts, and you can mix up a different salad combination every day. A little planning and you're good to go!

Pump Some Iron

You must exercise or melting the sweet potatoes drowned in marshmallows off your ass will take centuries.

If you're like me, meetings take over your calendar and evening social events leave you no time for the gym, just schedule your gym time on your calendar, as it's the most important thing you do each day. This is the one meeting that doesn't involve listening to droning voices at a roundtable topped with coffee and donuts and cookies galore. This meeting is one with yourself— it can't be rescheduled because your health is your number one priority. Who would reschedule that?!

Get exercise while being social. When I'm trying to compensate for bad eating behavior, I limit my dinner invitation acceptances and instead I make plans with my friends to do a gym class with them or go for a long walk to catch up. When you're chatting about who's cheating on whom, the time just flies by. Who knew gossip was the next best diet?

Music also makes it better. Update your iPod or make a new YouTube playlist. Listening to great tunes will motivate you to get more from your workouts or even keep you doing jumping jacks at home longer. Hip-hop and R&B are my jams of choice. Songs from Jay-Z, Rihanna, Beyoncé, Mario, Ne-Yo, and the Black Eyed Peas get my heart rate up. Sorry, folks, no "Party in the USA" Miley Cyrus stuff for me. Hip-hop gets me in the zone, not to mention I get to show off my uncanny ability to remember lyrics. Speaking of music, Britney Spears is a model example of the morning after. She went from rock-hard abs to baby body to too many trips to Starbucks, making her a tub of love, back to abs of steel for her Circus tour. Oops, she did it again. Same goes for you; with a bit of discipline and a lot of confidence you can make lasting changes to your life. So, take a look in the mirror and give thanks for what you've got.

Now, you have 364 days to start working out your body before the fattest day of the year. In the meantime, start treadmilling that turkey away!

YOU CAN'T MAKE THIS STUFF UP

Chapter 16

Liar, Liar, Plate on Fire

Diet and Nutrition Myths Debunked

As far as the old adage "finish everything on your plate" goes, I do rebut, although 27 percent of us finish everything on our plate even when we're full. Eat till you are full and then smile, have a conversation, but avoid mindless eating. When it comes to dieting, do your research. Diet myths help sell tween magazines. I am past that stage—for sure.

Working on Fifth Avenue right around the corner from all those fancy fashion week shows, I do get my share of being a spectator for Carlos Miele, Zac Posen, DVF, and other glammed-up shows with those size zeros strutting in a queue. I sure know they didn't go to zero by sticking to a well-balanced diet. So I will share with you my findings on non-facts. It's time to reveal the dieting magazines' betrayal, because not knowing the truth can be hazardous to your health.

Carbs

First and foremost, let's talk about carbs. Gals, when you need to eat pasta, please go right ahead. Just ask for the whole wheat variety and, if you can, stick to a fresh marinara and you'll be set. A cup of whole-grain pasta has the same amount of calories as white pasta, but of course, the whole-grain one is better. It's the cream and carbs, the heavy red meat and carbs, the BUTTER and carbs that will have you buying Spanx like they are Kleenex. Moderation, loveys, learn it!

I have read many low-carb diet books. My thoughts? Tempting, but tricky. You see, gals, living on just yogurt, fruit, nuts, and sex, the obvious, might seem like a great idea, but it's not really sustainable.

Low-carb diets don't actually provide enough fuel for your daily routine. Therefore your body goes into crisis mode and begins to delve into the stored carbs bin or glycogen for energy. When your body burns the stored carbs, water is released. This is the equivalent of taking water pills from your local drugstore. DON'T do it!

Those low-rise jeans that came out after the year 2000, yes, bellies popped because gals didn't control their diets accordingly. No extra length in the rise to hold in the muffin top. Beware of the tires . . . they roll right on in; it's only a matter of time. Still, avoiding carbs is not the answer.

Skipping Meals

In this chaotic world we live in today, ads for Pizza Hut pop into your living room when you are doing sits-ups in front of the sofa, and e-mail messages from Fresh Direct selling lobster ravioli in a pink creamy sauce appear instantly in your inbox. Your mind races, your tummy growls, and you get up and look feverishly for a snack. Depends on what's around—it could be anything, as you skipped lunch, but you shall pay for it in calories.

Lack of fueling your vehicle may result in an accident. Ladies, don't let this happen to you. Eat every few hours; that way you get time to plan, tabulate, and make better choices. When you skip a meal, you end up sending your body into starvation mode, which in effect makes you eat a whole lot more that you would otherwise. Try and go for less salt, drink more water, and eat fruit. I know it sounds odd but it's true. I never miss a meal. I eat three a day, plus usually two snacks. At 4:00 P.M. my tummy growls at my desk and I reach for some Driscoll's berries. It's a game, how are you going to play it? Skipping meals is for head-ache lovers.

Sugar—Brown, White, Organic??

This is hard to believe, but it doesn't matter. You see that divided box at Starbucks? There are sachets in all colors of the rainbow. Pink, blue, brown, white. The fancy European cafés have the long skinny packets in multicolors. Sugar lovers, pay attention. Most brown sugar on the shelves is actually white sugar colored with molasses. Don't go by the packaging, guys. Read the labels.

Shocked? Don't be. There's more. Brown sugar does have benefits; there are added minerals. But those minerals need to be eaten in large portions to have a positive effect in your system. So technically, brown and white sugar are essentially the same. I prefer brown just for the taste. Just tread cautiously when adding sugar to your food or beverage. There are really no gaping differences between the two.

Beef, Lamb, and Other Animals on Four Legs

Half of my family is vegetarian. The other half can't live without a butterfly filet mignon in garlic. Each birthday celebration becomes a weeklong discussion of the menu options at a few select eateries so that we can make sure to please everyone. It's a rather painful topic.

I, too, have spent a couple of year stints cleansing my system by being vegetarian and going for the green stuff. But at the end of the day, when I smell lamb chops or a yummy Bolognese, I go grab a plate. Being around chefs each day, I have to try new things. I have eaten undercooked partridge and have chowed down on steak at 9:30 A.M. Basically, I have to do what flows on camera. Therefore, I can't really be uber picky. I have, however, done some of my own investigating into the matter. Red meat provides a constant source of energy and essential amino acids that our bodies require. Each forkful of steak au poivre contains iron and phosphorus, which are far more easily digested and absorbed in our systems than what is found in grains and legumes. If you are afraid of red meat, don't be. It's really about the cuts. Just imagine what pork belly will look like on your belly. You get my point.

I personally go for hormone-free, organic lean cuts. Red meat can be high in saturated fats, similar to chicken with the skin on. So take your pick. Keep in mind that preserved meats like ham, bacon, and salami should be purchased carefully. Most producers add salt and nitrates, which are known to be carcinogenic. Go for the fresh stuff. Put on your cozy sweats and run out for some fresh, lean cuts that are the real thing, not sitting in plastic for weeks and weeks.

Bad Fat? Good Fat?

While we are talking about the fatty stuff, let's debunk the mystery on this topic. Fat sure does make you fat. It's definitely harder to fit into your skinny jeans. Thank heavens for J Brand—everyone needs a little leeway. It's truly a matter of good fats vs. bad fats. In simple terms, avocados vs. lard. You get the visual?

Bad fats are known as saturated or trans fats. These are cholesterol promoting and bad for your cardiac health. When I was at Goldman Sachs back in the day, I used to put a caution sign up each time a pal would eat a cheeseburger. Mind you, he did this about four to five times a week. That could cause some heart trouble. There isn't a cardio workout on the planet that can save you from an uber-atty diet. This I realized at the ripe age of thirty. It got me thinking, but I never stopped eating. I just made better choices.

Good fats are monounsaturated and polyunsaturated. Examples include nuts, olives, and avocados. These manage to raise the level of good cholesterol in your system while reducing the level of bad. Bring it down to your everyday salad. A few slices of avocado or a sprinkle of almond slivers sure beat the nutritional value of bacon bits while providing great texture and flavor. When making dinner or even a dressing for a salad, opt for olive oil.

While some fats are better than others, the fat cell doesn't know the difference between a good fat and a bad fat. All excess calories, whether they are good fats, bad fats, protein, or carbs, will be stored as body fat, so please, consume all fats in moderation.

Easy enough. If you want to balance in those 5½-inch heels at RDV, then you've got to embrace a balanced diet. A slender waist never photographed poorly.

Five Foods That Have More Calories Than You Think

It's no surprise that many restaurants sugarcoat more than their dessert menus. But don't let other not-so-sugary meals fool you, either. Once you take in more calories than your body weight calls for, those excess calories turn to excess fat. Don't let flavor fool you. Food can be quite talented at fraud these days.

1. *Trail mix:* Sure, it starts with almonds, raisins, and dried fruit, but it's easy for popular brands to slip in things like heavily salted peanuts, M&Ms and oily banana chips. Although they seem healthy, some trail mixes can have as many as 693 calories per serving! Trader Joe's Omega Trail Mix has 170 calories per serving (about one cup), but we all know that measuring out a single cup is doubtful when you're on a snacking binge. Instead, by making yourself a simple turkey sandwich on whole-wheat bread with some veggies, you'll feel full for longer, and on fewer calories..

2. *Coconut:* Just because it's a fruit does not mean it's low in calories. One serving of 50 grams of fresh coconut already has 180 calories. And it doesn't stop there—other coconut dishes such as Thai coconut soup can have more than 300 calories, while coconut milk can pack up to 450 calories per cup! If you really crave the coconut, stick to fresh slices or coconut frozen fruit bars, which are under the 200-calorie count.

Even better, try hydrating with coconut water, which is rich in potassium and electrolytes.

3. *Salad:* Although this secret has been out of the bag for a while, people still like to pretend that ordering a salad when dining out means they are being "good" for the night, whatever that means. So keep pretending that your buffalo ranch chicken salad is healthy just because it's served over a bed of greens, or face reality and come to terms with the fact that you could order a single milkshake and still consume fewer calories than your salad. Panera's BBQ chicken chopped salad, for example, is 500 calories. And if I got into the calorie portion of some Caesar salads, you might fall over. Two tablespoons of Caesar dressing alone is about 170 calories. You can have a whole-wheat mini bagel and almond butter for about the same amount. So do yourself a favor and pass up salads that include bacon, cheese, ham, prosciutto, and other nonsense—or even better, save the salad for home. Then you can add and measure out your own toppings. Dip your fork into a cup of dressing each time you take a bite of salad. You'll still get the flavor without dousing your salad with about 200 calories' worth of oily, creamy crap.

4. *Peanut butter:* Sometimes I feel like the official spokesman for almond butter. Its main competition, peanut butter, comes in at 210 calories per serving. Even two tablespoons of Green Ways Organic Creamy Peanut butter has 200 calories, so don't let the "O" word fool you. Peanut butter may be packed with protein, but so are a lot of other options that won't jack up the calorie count.

5. *Guacamole:* I'm all for avocados—they are among my super foods. But when you mix this healthy fat with cilantro, onions, tomatoes, lime juice, and the rest of the Mexican medley to make guacamole, this super food can turn deadly. One serving of guacamole, ¼ cup, is 360 calories. Avocados are what make guacamole so high in calories, and once you serve it with corn chips, then throw in some margaritas, you've got yourself almost an entire day's worth of calories.

Egg-tastic

Yes, eggs are fantastic. I was raised on eggs—hard boiled, scrambled with cheese, or in frittatas. My mom doesn't love yolks but in summary—we are an egg-loving family. Minus my nephews, of course, who have recently discovered buckwheat pancakes with REAL maple syrup and think egg yolks are "yucky." It's only a matter of time till they discover the goodness of the essential amino acids.

Shopping for eggs has become rather confusing. Aside from either paying $3.00 for a dozen or $6.79, what really matters when you're shopping for eggs? Brown vs. white? Organic or regular? Cage free? Omega-3 enhanced? I get a migraine thinking about the options. Marketers had me on this one for a while. I had to buzz my nutritionist friends for some further insight. This is what I found:

The nutrition in brown vs. white eggs is the same. The color of the shell comes from the breed of the hen. Figure that out! So go certified organic if you are concerned about hormones and antibiotics. It is pretty logical. But all the images and colors can certainly throw you off. It's like going down the cereal aisle. The junk definitely looks better dressed than the healthy alternatives.

The cage-free signage relates to the animal welfare or treatment of the hens. That, too, is a personal choice. If you can afford it, it's yours. Always read the labels. That goes for anything and everything you are purchasing.

As for omega-3 fortified, research has determined that these eggs have health benefits up to seven times more than regular eggs. The good news is you don't have to go to Whole Foods for these products. Every grocery now carries the full assortment. So start your day with a healthy omelet and you'll sustain energy and brain power till happy hour.

Pills and Cleanses

Losing weight is hard. Staying slim and fit is hard. Taking diet pills and doing cleanses is easy. So here's a hard lesson in life: taking the easy way out never works. Yup, you heard it here first. You can get quick results from gimmicks, fasts, pills, and diets, but if you want to respect your body for the gorgeous temple it is and make real changes that will help your long-term health, you need to do it the hard way. Every girl flirts with diet pills and has a fling with the body cleanse of the month, but truth be told, we are all better off going steady with our sneakers. After working on a deal and being glued to my desk at work for months, I got desperate and took a dive into diet pill land. I bought Alli and took about half the dosage suggested. Aside from making the stinkiest farts and craps of my life, I was completely grossed out by the oil drops in the toilet bowl (the fat that wasn't being digested by my body). But it gets better: my stomach was constantly in knots and on one particular summer day I couldn't stop farting all day. I also had a date that night and I was nervous. Anyhow, I went to the restaurant and sat down on a chair in the lounge. The hostess walked over to me minutes later and called me aside. She whispered in my ear, "I think you pooped in your pants. You might want to hit the bathroom." My heart sank and, sure enough, I had to take off my white Theory pants and wash them frantically in the sink. What I thought was a stinky bad fart was actually a watery poop. Thank god for individual bathrooms and also for hand dryers. I had an orange-colored stain on my pants that I couldn't get rid of, but luckily I was back in action at the bar after five minutes of hand-drying my white pants. Lesson learned. No diet pills for me—EVER again. Talk about embarrassing side effects . . .

Nutrition myths have controlled our diets for years. Don't eat this because . . . this color sugar is bad because . . . Enough is enough! If half of these myths were true, we would all starve to death trying to make the right choices.

When it comes to food, most of the "facts" you hear are not facts at all (unless your reading them off of a Snapple cap, of course). So do not feed into the bullshit of food myths. By now you're way past Santa Claus and the Tooth Fairy. I think you should also be way past eggshell colors and cancer-causing snacks, and do some research instead of relying on the overflowing mouths of others. Instead of always eating, do a little reading, so you, and only you, know what's best for your body.

Don't . . .

- ➤ Ax carbs from your diet
- ➤ Skip meals (EVER!)

- Think eating brown sugar is better for you than white sugar
- Be afraid of red meat. Chose wisely and avoid sodium and chemicals
- Be fooled that brown eggs are better than white ones
- Take the easy way out, relying on diet pills and cleanses to keep your weight in control

411 on Shakes and Protein Powder

Ladies, let me be clear: I don't encourage drinking protein shakes or powders, and it's even worse to skip a meal altogether and end up stuffing your face later in the day, but we all know some days you just have to power through with something fast and filling. Here's the skinny on the shakes, powders, and juices that are out there to choose from:

1. *Spiru-Tein:* If you're shooting for taste, this protein powder takes the cake (or should I say "shake?"). Chock-full of essential nutrients and soy protein, this 100-percent vegan protein powder also contains hearty doses of fiber to keep you feeling full. The only downside? Unless you want clumping, you'll need a blender to mix this powder with your choice of milk, soy milk, or juice. GNC sells these awesome "blender bottles." I have one. (No, I'm not crazy, I swear.)

2. *Slimfast:* Nothing controls calories better than one of these premade shakes, which only contain 200 calories a pop . . . not bad considering each can contains 15 grams of protein. But beware, the main three ingredients in these chocolatey sweet shakes are skim milk, fructose, and cocoa—in other words, 35 grams of sugar. Remember, high sugar intake often leads to cravings and an increased appetite later on.

3. *Naked Protein Zone Juices:* These protein-enriched juices top the charts with a whopping 30 grams of protein in each bottle. They aren't exactly low in cholesterol (30 mg per bottle) or sodium (140 mg), but the good news is that they are made from all-natural, easy to pronounce ingredients and pure soy protein.

The moral of the story? As long as you opt for a high-protein, low-sugar powder or shake, protein supplements can be perfectly acceptable substitutes for those days when you don't have time to cook. Just don't make a habit of it!

Chapter 17

Spot Secret

My Name Is Divya and I'm a Spillaholic

I got glasses in the third grade. I remember being nervous about wearing them in Ms. Gladstone's class. I was fearful of the typical four-eyed freak names the "cool" kids would call me. Luckily, I got over that fear when I became the cool kid with the glasses. This not-so-invisible best friend of a frame became permanently attached to my hip, or should I say, face. At night I would sleep with my glasses on. My mom would remove them in the middle of the night (she's lucky I never woke up) and then ask me in the morning, "Why do you wear your glasses to bed?" I replied, "So I can see my dreams clearly." Clearly, I was a genius child. Unfortunately, this was not my only bad bedtime habit. I also chewed gum like a cow with horrible manners (according to my dad) and fell asleep with it in my mouth. No, I never choked, but an hour of peanut butter and haircomb action usually ensued when I woke up.

I came home from every kid's birthday party a guilty suspect. I didn't steal the cookie from the cookie jar . . . ha, I was way more daring. I was a total pizza hoarder, often with a nice big greasy spot on my T-shirt or shorts, not to mention a few drops of mint chocolate-chip ice cream on my poor choice of a white T-shirt.

Now as a culinary media entrepreneur, I eat, all day, every day. Think Samantha from *Sex and the City*; her with sex, is me with food . . . trust me, if I could switch roles for a day I would. Yet, just like Samantha Jones is a sex goddess, I, Divya Gugnani, am a goddess in many culinary ways. One of my areas of expertise has become stain removal. I have the healing touch—for fabric at least (if only it would also apply to men!). We didn't call this book a black book for nothing. It's damn useful to know how to get spills out before they set. Especially when you're like me, borrowing clothes from designers for filming and don't want to have your tail between your legs when it comes time to returning soiled garments to Jay Godfrey, Ankasa, and many others.

Numero uno: blot before you begin. A clean towel or dishrag should be applied directly on the dirty spot to remove any excess food, grease, or foreign particles that appear on your wardrobe.

Dish soap does more than dishes—it's been around the block, or I guess sink, if you get my point. Applied with a little water and some help from an old toothbrush, it can hide the drips of grease that got away from your fork. Salad dressing decides to land on your shirt cuff? Dish soap will do the trick. Mac and cheese make its way onto your button-down? Try this remedy. The greasier the stain, the more high-powered dish soap you will need. To the cleaning lady that replenishes our stock in our office kitchen, no we're not washing dishes, no we're not eating it, but we're sure using it to clean our clothes. Dish soap will do anything, and maybe anyone, yet it's still clean . . . amazing! Protein shampoo has similar effects, so try it if you're fresh out of dish soap.

Boil it out. While discussing the benefit of tea on a recent shoot, Earl Grey decided to make a nice little scorching design on my brand-new outfit. Since I'm not a regular tea drinker, I was stumped. But a lightbulb went off in my brain (I guess it was the caffeine): boiling water. I submerged the stains with super-hot water and the tea faded before my eyes. At times I've used this trick for berries, with modest success. I've shared it with my Starbucks addict friends who claim it works like a charm for their morning mishaps of spilling coffee on the go.

Sunlight for spices. The term "spice" originated way before the annoying Spice Girls hit the charts—even though some people think differently. In fact, even without this teenybopper girl band, spices have been enhancing restaurant menus and dinner parties alike these days. Chef Marcus Samuelsson is a particular offender who comes to mind in this department. He always uses African and Indian spices to ignite flavor in his food. Love the smell, buddy, but hate the stain. I'd much rather it caused a fire in my mouth than a yellow sun shape on my pants—the shit was impossible to get out, until I discovered the power of sunlight. Sure, it helps plants grow and keeps this Earth alive. But most important, it does wonders on my clothes. Instead of scrubbing and fussing with spice stains (which usually only makes them yellow), I place the garment outside to allow Mother Nature to brighten up our day and take those despised stains away.

White wine vinegar is much more than a salad dressing, let

me tell you. On a recent trip to Spain, I ate my way through Asturias, stopping along the way to film episodes of our show, and drink tempranillo and garnacha. As luck would have it, my tapas and fragrant entrées had a reddish tinge from cayenne peppers that spiced their way on to my daily dresses. Since dish soap couldn't battle it alone, I learned it was best to run cold water over the stain, scrub with dish soap, and then add white wine vinegar diluted in water to finish things off. White wine vinegar is my new holy water, saving my dresses from disgrace.

Baby powder doesn't just disguise dirty hair. We've all done the "I didn't have time to wash my hair so I dumped a bunch of baby powder on my head to soak up the oil in my greasy roots," but I'm going to do you one better. Arrabbiata sauce overboard? Joey Campanaro's creamy risotto at The Little Owl leave its mark? Apply a lot of baby powder to a greasy stain (especially if the fabric is silk) and shake off the excess. Repeat a few times if necessary. Once you think the baby powder has sucked up all the grease, shake some more on there and let it sit for a few minutes, just for good measure. Now you see a big white spot on your clothes. Do not fret, rub the white spot (covered in baby powder) against another nonstained section of your item and you should be grease free. Now go put a little baby powder under those armpits. You have been schvitzing, trying to get out the stain. Note: cornstarch (for those of us who actually cook at home) can work the same magic as baby powder.

Put a Spell on Your Spills: Wine Stain Remedies

We all know wine is our best friend when it comes to candle-lit dinners, an urge for a nice sleepy drunk, or a girls'-night over chick flicks and spinach dip. Yet I plead guilty to being a bi-polar bitch once that lovely bottle of red wine hits my rug, or even better, my favorite shirt that just happens to be borrowed from my best friend's closet (whoops!). Now wine is no longer on my good side. As a wine lover, wine stains are a common part of my everyday life—lucky me! Yet I've learned some simple tac-tics to tackle the consequences of my next wine-stained cocktail dress. First of all, people, OxiClean works wonders. You can buy it anywhere. Just spray several times where the wine is located, let dry for about a half hour, and throw it in the wash. No one will ever know—especially the owner of the outfit (which clearly wasn't me during my first encounter).

For people who enjoy directions, follow a more structured technique, rather than whining about your wine-spotted clothes:

1. Blot the stain immediately with paper towels. If it is a dry-clean-only garment, do not do anything, and don't pretend you're some wizard in the stain field. Instead, march that fabric's ass straight to the cleaners if you ever want to see the outfit in your closet again. Pretreatment of the stain may cause permanent damage and the dry cleaner may not be able to remove the stain (they are not all miracle workers).

2. Combine 1 teaspoon of detergent and 1 cup of hydrogen per-oxide in a small bowl. Soak a clean sponge in the mixture, wring it halfway dry, and then gently blot the stain.

3. We never want to stain more than what is already stained (obviously), unless, of course, you're looking for an excuse to throw out Grandma's apple green sweater vest given to you last Christmas. But if it is not a sweater vest, place a dry towel

between the front and back of the garment as long as the stain has not penetrated through to the back of the fabric. This will prevent staining the opposite side of the material.

4. If, and only if, the fabric is machine washable (we can all read labels), wash in cool water and air dry. If the fabric is hand wash only, wash gently in the sink with a mild detergent.

Chocolate Catastrophes

We don't have to be five years old to be victims of chocolate stains. I, for one, am chocolate obsessed. Dark, light, rich, sweet, and moist—I like it all (and no, I am not talking about men . . . but I could be!). Anyhow, chocolate is as much of a vice to me as it is to my clothes. Here's what I do:

1. Always allow melted chocolate to dry and harden. Many mindless chocolate lovers think using a wet paper towel on melted chocolate does some sort of magic until they realize it is an epic fail. The chocolate will smudge and provide even more damage to that lovely white summer dress. The stain's already on you, so waiting a little longer for it to dry won't kill you—it'll just make more people realize how much of a slob you are.

2. Next, scrape away hardened chocolate with blunt knife. Be sure not to stab yourself. This isn't an attempt to visit the nearest emergency room and get off work for a week (I know, the temptation!). Focus only on the hard chocolate to also avoid poking any holes in your clothing. You're removing the stain to rewear the clothes, right?

3. Finally, pretreat the stain with stain remover—I prefer Stain Stick—or detergent and wash as directed by its label. Oh, and I'd lay off chocolate for the rest of the evening. Tomorrow's a brand-new day, eager and ready to tackle those stains.

The Answer Is, Simply, Club Soda

Did you know substituting club soda for the liquid called for in many recipes enhances the fluffiness of pancakes and waffles? Or that the minerals in the soda water help green plants grow? For best results, try to water your plants with club soda about once a week. If you love oysters but find shucking them to be a near-impossible chore, try soaking them in club soda before you shuck. The oysters will be much easier to open. Soak your diamonds, rubies, sapphires, and emeralds in club soda—this allows you to tell the little white lie, "Oh they're brand new, just a silly little gift from my hubby." Simply place your jewels in a glass full of club soda and let them soak overnight. Cold club soda with a dash of bitters even works wonders on an upset stomach.

I hope you didn't think club soda could do all this and not be an expert at stain removal (I feel like I'm advertising on some infomercial with this item!).

But yes, club soda allows you to clean grease stains from double-knit fabrics. Pour club soda on the stain and scrub gently. Scrub more vigorously to remove stains on carpets or less delicate articles of clothing. It even cleans the crap off your windshield—literally. Keep a spray bottle filled with club soda in the trunk of your car. Use it to help remove bird droppings and greasy stains from the windshield.

Oh, and don't spend money on pointless cleaners like Mr.

Clean, Pledge, or the "miraculous Swiffer Sweeper" (miraculous, my ass!). Instead, pour club soda directly on stainless steel countertops, ranges, and sinks. Wipe with a soft cloth, rinse with warm water, and wipe dry. To clean porcelain fixtures, simply pour club soda over them and wipe with a soft cloth. There's no need for soap or rinsing, and the soda will not mar the finish. Give the inside of your refrigerator a good cleaning with a weak solution of club soda and a little bit of salt.

Finally, it also makes the post-dinner cleanup an effortless task. Food tastes delicious when it's cooked in cast iron, if you're willing to do the dirty work, and I'm not talking Sopranos-style hit man here. This work is way worse: the cleaning, the agony of those heavy pots and pans with the sticky mess inside that makes you wish magic really did exist. You can make the cleanup a lot easier by pouring some club soda in the pan while it's still warm. The bubbly soda will keep the mess from sticking and your hands in a lot less stress.

As Dirty as a Baby's Bottom

My sister, mother of two naughty boys, has abandoned the use of clutch bags, as they are not mom-friendly. Every time I see her I notice two things. 1. She looks more tired than she did the last time (proof that those boys are sure giving her a run for her money). 2. Her handbag gets bigger. It's filled with "mommy stuff," she says. Mommies know best (just as she did with breakfast), as her baby wipes have rescued lipstick that stained my chin after eating Sergio Bitici's bucatini alla matriciana, eye shadow that hit my pants during a session with Dr. Stephen Gullo about drinking on a diet, and mascara slips that are left best off my forehead.

Cold Water Cures

For those unexpected days when your period decides to pay you a visit or when you walk into a table while delivering opening lines and have a knee gushing with blood, take off the soiled victim and submerge it in cold water immediately. The sooner you do it, the more likely you are to erase any trace of the blood bath, and attract more people in your personal proximity.

Yet I cannot always cure all red stains. Tomatoes are tough. A lover of all things Italian, I've learned tomatoes are very tricky and best left to the professional, the god of all stain removers, the dry cleaner. Besides, it'll be a rare visit, since you just cut your dry-cleaning bill in half with these tips. One trip to the cleaner's for tomato stains won't hurt. If anything, it'll keep them from going out of business.

Chapter 18

How Not to Be a Heifer This Holiday

Only Santa Should Be Fat on Christmas

I think I've always been "that girl." No, not the drunken sloppy one, grinding with co-workers to 80's tunes at her company holiday party. Not the one who wears too short a skirt to church. Not the one who's always late and keeps her friends waiting. I'm the girl who has a bit too much good taste—and by taste, I don't mean the latest Dolce and Gabbana dress.

During the holidays, most people discover a new addiction to shopping. Christmas is the perfect excuse to buy your best friend Chanel perfume, and then accidentally pick up an extra one for yourself. Unfortunately, my holiday addiction is not about smelling good. Instead, it's about what tastes good. My addiction is food.

I discovered early on that the holiday buffet would soon re-place any pair of shoes as my new best friend. It all started when my friend Alba, an event planner in New York City, invited me to the *Dreamgirls* movie premiere. Imagine me, up close and personal with Beyoncé, Eddie Murphy, Jennifer Hudson, along with the other movie stars . . . every girl's dream, right? Well, while my other friends practically fainted from star-struck syndrome, I found myself away from all the Hollywood hype, landing a cozy spot right next to the buffet. Surprised at all?

From then on, whenever I attended some glamorous event, the question "Where's Divya?" was always answered by the chronic response "She's wherever the buffet is," which became a pointless question after my regular habit became widespread knowledge. I'd rather eat my calories than drink them. Put it this way: if I were at the Grammys, I'd be more interested in cream puffs than I'd be in Puff Daddy . . . pathetic, I know.

But as the years have gone on, and Facebook friends now outnumber my address book contacts, the holiday cocktail party invites have only increased—only now RSVPing is as easy as the click of a mouse rather than the tiresome stamp-placing, envelope-licking, anthrax infecting mailing process. On Facebook, clicking on "attending" takes no time at all. So how could I resist? After my first year of the holiday glitz and a size up in my Mrs. Claus costume for a themed party, I soon realized the buffet was the exact place I should not be.

With so many tasty events, I'm always so tempted to make about five trips back to the buffet bar. But the holidays are also a great time to stay fit and fabulously tempted. All you need is some control, although control is never easy. So, I took some time to create a strategy for these never-ending cherry cheesecake–packed events. Now I want to share my game plan with you (you're welcome in advance).

First off, whenever I go to a party, I leave the office twenty to thirty minutes early, in flats, of course—I haven't reached the status warranting a personal driver. Cabbing it is called laziness—you might as well have someone dress you in the morning if you can't even walk your fat ass a few extra blocks. Without a car, I can take my time to walk (or stride) to the event and pull the good old heel switcheroo out of my plastic grocery bags. Bystanders think I went shopping, while I secretly get my twenty-minute exercise in on a cold December evening . . . genius, I know. Plus, the walking always gives me an extra boost of energy before I enter the party, which doesn't hurt when you're still secretly searching for a potential soul mate.

The second plan is hydration. I always drink a lot of water before I go. It keeps me full. Drink enough water to quench your thirst daily. This will serve as good motivation for fitting into that cute little black dress that looks brand new, even though you bought it two years ago. Who has time to shop for a different holiday outfit every night of the week? I did that in middle school for the endless year of themed bat mitzvahs . . . I refuse to do it again.

Okay, now comes the game plan for alcohol. We all know it's hard to resist the luscious holiday candy-cane martini cocktail— that was until I found out the majority of them were 200 to 300 calories, not to mention they put you in a sugar shock. One cocktail once in a while is fine. But for the majority of your nights, opt for red wine. Even better, mixing half a glass of red wine with club soda or sparkling water will cut your calories in half . . . and it's actually more refreshing than that chocolate-peppermint martini that just made you wish you could unbutton your pants for a second. Come on, ladies, we've all been there. I personally love club soda with a splash of cranberry or lime juice. It gives me a boost of vitamin C, and by not drinking the alcohol, I'll have enough sense in me to leave the party whenever I want. Trust me, sometimes when you're at parties hosted by your lawyer or your ex-boyfriend's best friend who your best friend happens to be dating now—you want to be able to think straight. Your one focus: grab a pig-in-a-blanket and bounce.

For the parties you do want to stick around for, I always try to eat a little before I go so I'm partially satisfied when I arrive. You also do not want to skip any meals the day of the event. Trust me, I've done the whole "let me not eat today so I have an excuse to stuff my face in fried shrimp and pudding tonight!" Well, this had to be even dumber than the time I thought walking while eating a bagel made the cream cheese lower in fat (yes, I did go to both Cornell and Harvard, lapse of intelligence, that's all). By not eating before a party, you are only tempted to go there and overgorge like it's the Last Supper, only Christ is replaced by Santa Claus. But if you do eat a little, you'll be hungry for small snacks, such as the veggie platter—celery, carrots, cucumbers, and cauliflower are almost always offered. Just put the dip on the side and tread with caution! But please, please, do not be the person who finished the entire portion of celery before eight o'clock. You'll look like a starving bunny rabbit and get green stuff in between your teeth. And don't indulge in some garlicky tomato dipping oil either. You never know when there'll be mistletoe around. Unless, of course, you walk under it simultaneously with the seventeen-year-old Steve Urkle lookalike McDonald's cashier who snuck into the Ritz-Carlton on a dare from his buddies. I hope that's the night you ate the garlic.

When it comes to the meat samplers, avoid all the fried bites.

We all know what it tastes like. If you don't, take a nibble. Stick to the good protein—turkey without the bread or hamburgers without the buns. Sometimes people look at me like I'm crazy, but every little bit counts. I've had more sandwiches and cheeseburgers than you can imagine. I founded a culinary media brand focused on tips, tricks, and techniques for God's sake. Will I die without having one more at this party? No. I've learned that the more you eat, the more you must take off. Why make life harder than it has to be? Let taxes and clogged toilet drains be your life crises, not a weight gain every time Thanksgiving rolls around.

Healthy snacks at work will help you stay full too (see Table, Smart Snacking, p. 102). The most important thing to do before you leave is take a good look at yourself in the mirror. If you look fabulous, unless it's some sort of bad-hair day because your blow-dryer burned out, you'll want to stay looking fabulous all night. You must make that mind-body connection of "I want to look fabulous, and I will." If you think this way, you will look this way. Fab is the way to be, so make it part of your vocabulary.

However, there is one thing I never do. I do not go to a party without eating dessert. Sorry folks, can't do it. And why should I? I'm not saying I scarf down a whole peanut butter chocolate mousse pie all by myself . . . even though I could. Instead, I taste everything. Tasting and eating are two very different concepts. When I taste, I still enjoy every dessert offered without feeling guilt in my gut. But don't beat yourself up if you decide to have two cookies one night or a whole slice of marble loaf. So what? Just don't do it all the time. Life is about moderation. The extra cocktail or the extra dessert every single time won't do you any better the next day. So why bother?

And finally, the key to staying fit, and the most essential component of every party, is the dance floor. Now, instead of the buffet, you can always find me there. I dance like the DJ is always playing my song, and my song is not Lady Gaga's "Just Dance." I've been doing this act way before her time. Not only does dancing allow me to show off my talented moves, but it keeps me away from the buffet and allows me to burn off that cheese chunk and cracker I just gobbled down. Even if there's only one grumpy old man on the floor, I dance. I couldn't care less. It's fun! And the dance party doesn't stop there. When I go out at night, I always continue the party at home. I get my iTunes play list of hip-hop big pimpin' songs (wouldn't have it any other way), and I dance. Other times, I fire up my Mac and get busy to my YouTube playlist of upbeat songs. The party never ends for me, even if it's at 3:00 A.M. and I have to catch an 8:00 A.M. train. Every dancing session just gets me ready for the slim chance that I'll be able to bust out my skills on the revival of *Soul Train*.

I even make sure my dinner parties turn into dance parties. Fortunately, I've found a new love. Sorry, buffet, but my dancing shoes have kicked your calorie-filled stomach-stuffing platters to the curb.

Chapter 19

A Mano Is Not a Man

Ladies, Don't Date a Man Who Won't Eat a Meal

Before I could shed a tear after my final breakup with Mr. Greenwich, Mr. M asked me out to dinner. We'd been friends for a year and were both young, energetic entrepreneurs, so I thought, "Why not?" and we went for it. Our conversation was heated. He asked me out religiously once a week and took a good twenty-four to forty-eight hours to respond to my e-mails. Talk about playing hard to get . . .

Week four, when our first kiss was yet to come, I began to wonder if he was gay. Was it my apple-bottom butt that was preventing him from making a move? In fact, I pulled out all the stops and channeled the culinary goddess in me, preparing an elaborate three-course meal at my apartment. I composed a beet salad with goat cheese and candied walnuts, Asian salmon marinated in soy and sesame oil, and a dessert of berries and fresh vanilla whipped cream. Surely my cooking could seduce anyone with an appetite, I thought. But lucky me, I didn't even get a peck. Was he just intimidated by my cooking expertise?

Then, after I motivated myself to go on a blind date (couldn't get much worse than dating a noneater), a text arrived from Mr. M, "Let's meet up for a drink." I wondered . . . hmm . . . I just saw him for our weekly three-hour meal, why was he throwing me a curve ball? (Clearly, meatballs were not his style.) Sure enough, that night was the beginning of our romantic relationship.

We confided in each other about our work struggles: hiring, firing, building technology platforms, and lots of other oh so romantic stuff in the corporate world, of course. Our friendship was a strong one, but it was meals that were our rough spot. I would order and polish off everything on my plate like a good girl. He, however, would move his food from side to side without ingesting very much. Then it struck me. He'd lost a good thirty pounds in the last year and seemed to have a difficult relationship with food, whereas my relationship with food was a happy, healthy one. Well, healthy is questionable depending on the dessert menu. I don't eat to live; rather, I live to eat. I enjoy each and every savory or sweet bite as my palate explodes with joy and gratitude.

Mr. M kept a food journal and constantly punished himself for slight missteps of mild overeating or unhealthy eating. His relationship with his body was equally abusive. He ran miles on end trying to make amends for the moderate amounts of food that entered his system. I just didn't understand it, but I knew it was a sign of his emotionally troubled mental state.

Then one day he asked me to prepare all of his favorite dishes for a dinner party with another couple. I spent a good six hours preparing and cooking. When the guests arrived, I was only too pleased to see him devour everything on his plate and reach for seconds and thirds ("He's human!" I thought). We all headed to another party that my high school friend Amanda was hosting. He was fidgety and uncomfortable and stared at me restlessly most of the evening. He walked me to a cab and went home, telling me that he had to get up early to weigh in with his nutritionist and needed to get in a morning run before the session. I'm sorry, but who was the female in this relationship? He called me when he got home, feeling guilty about cutting our night short.

The next day after his meeting, he told me news that made me sick. Sadly, I wasn't the only one with the stomach trouble. He had gone home the prior night to force himself to vomit out all the food I had labored over cooking. He was afraid he wouldn't have reached his targeted weight loss for the week.

It was then that I realized I was in a relationship with a true manorexic. Sure, I'll admit that it bothered me that his stomach was flatter than mine, his abs had more definition, and he could drop ten pounds in less than two weeks, as if he was some magical Harry Potter weight wizard. But what bothered me more is that he made me edgy every time I took a bite of any meal. He'd order the fish and I'd be pigging out on lamb chops. He would look at me like I was Ms. Piggy, and he didn't want to be Kermit the Frog anymore. I felt like I was an overweight teenager with acne. It was beyond disturbing. Let's be honest, when has food ever come between me and anything, especially another person? Never! It usually mends the heartache and comforts the soul. This time it did the exact opposite.

My mother always told me to be comfortable in the skin I was in. Despite my strong will, Mr. M made me feel like a house, although I was eating like every other normal appetite holding woman. I stopped seeing Mr. M, and at our last meal together I smiled after I polished off my egg white omelet and he only finished half of his. I ran into him at a party many months later. We chatted and I politely told him that he was on my shit list (for more reasons than not just eating). He left the party with a tall blonde but, sure enough, I got a text at 1:45 A.M., "Let me know when I'm off your shit list so we can hang out." I responded, "Let me know what you are going to do to get off my shit list." He wrote back, "Come over and I'll show you." That required no response and wasn't even tempting for half a second.

So, ladies, always remember that the company you keep shapes how you feel inside and out. Never be with anyone who dulls your shine. Let the manorexics get therapy and attend classes on Women 101. Then find a real man who likes his meat— both on the ass and on the plate.

LIFE
LESSONS

Chapter 20

Office Space

Why Chocolate-Covered Cherries Are Not Lunch

Behind the Burner is brimming with food and drinks, both on and off the screen. It's no surprise that when working at a culinary media brand, your office is going to receive mounds and mounds of food. There are snacks galore in the kitchen, candy apples and chocolates during the holidays, enough wine to get an army drunk, not to mention the occasional turkey defrosting on our kitchen counter, and much, much more. I must say, the edible gifts are definitely a big perk of choosing a culinary career, as long as your half-hour lunch break doesn't consist of stuffing your face with free treats from the office pantry.

So, how does our staff stay slim and trim? We share the wealth! We sublet space from a law firm, which not only means intelligent, handsome men, but more important, large appetites!

Lawyers work late hours, as do we, but we leave our treats out for them to enjoy while we take off and hit the gym. It's like when little children leave cookies out for Santa and come back to find crumbs and a glass half full of milk (skim milk, of course). Only with us, we leave the goodies all year around, and it's much more than your average Toll-House.

Secondly, we keep treats in common areas. Never stash goodies in your desk. You'll find yourself munching on them mindlessly during conference calls and while writing e-mails—trust me, I've had that wonderful experience. Instead, keep them in a common area so you will have to get off your ass to eat one.

Regifting is mandatory. One person's garbage is another's gold. Take those Thanksgiving gift baskets, holiday cookies, and Valentine's Day chocolates and give them to your mailman, UPS delivery guy, hair stylist, roommate, or significant other (you don't want anyone else finding them attractive anyway). A little weight gain for these people won't hurt!

Another option is the terror of taking things home. If you decide to take this bold step, remember, the freezer is your friend. Freeze what you can and serve it to your dinner guests. I advise redistributing things into individual portions so you can create built-in control for yourself. For dessert nightmares, like chocolates or anything chocolate covered, I suggest keeping the tempting treats in a dark container and allowing them to hibernate for some time in a faraway cabinet. Studies have shown that we eat significantly more candy/sweets if they are placed in a clear container versus an opaque container. You're only allowed one treat per day, so just pretend you've forgotten where you stashed the prize until that sweet tooth starts aching a few hours after dinner. The agony no dentist could ever heal! If only they had candy insurance to pay for every cavity that sweets caused and to remove every pound our hips gained. Oh well, as a food lover, I can only dream of the possibilities to make life easy.

The holiday season doesn't have to be the only time to do a good deed (even though most people are lazy enough to believe that). Instead, make the homeless happy. We recently got a huge delivery of garlic to our office for a shoot. After dividing it among our staff, our families, and even our favorite chef friends, we had a huge box left. Garlic really does go a long way. It saved most of us money on seasoning our sauces and salads for months, and serves as an awesome remedy for the sore throats your average plain Jane green tea was definitely not tackling. Still, we were stuck with one final box of garlic. So we called local homeless shelters until we found someone to take our food, not to mention save us from the cause of all our bad breath.

If you can't tame your belly, get your ass out of the kitchen. If you know you won't have any self-control when presented with a spread of caramel popcorn, shortbread cookies, and chocolate-covered raisins, just keep them out of view and out of reach. I'm telling you, the kitchen is sometimes worse than revisiting old photos of former lovers. Not only will you suffer heartache from the weight gain that will appear on the scale in a week or so, but you'll also find yourself trapped again in a hopeless romance, full of bad habits and unhealthy ways. Instead, find a new partner for your mouth (I'm still talking food here). Bring your own fresh piece of fruit when going out or go for a walk to avoid the temptation. However, avoid walking to the nearest Starbucks and Chipotle, found on about every other street corner in New York. Fast food and sugar-induced caramel lattes are just as bad, if not worse, than our office snacks.

Fortunately, I am never too hard on myself because I did choose a career in food. Therefore, allow yourself one or two of your favorite holiday goodies a day, maybe 150 calories or 200 if you took the stairs to the office instead of the elevator. If your office is on the first floor, this does not count! Choose what you really want, eat it slowly, and enjoy it. Then stop! We humans have minds for many reasons. Self-control is one of them.

So, as I've discovered from the oh so yummy, yet dreadful edible gifts that visit my office every day, the best way to deal with gifts of food is to eat one, savor it, and then give the rest away. Besides, what's better than the gift of giving? But I must say, receiving doesn't hurt either!

Chapter 21

My Happy Pills

My Favorite Feel-Good Foods

I walk into work every day like the energizer bunny. Even on rainy days as I get smacked by tons of umbrellas through the wet streets of New York City, I always crack a smile. It's not because I like rain, or that I enjoy getting splashed by passing cars that decide to be assholes during the morning commute. It's days like these when my co-workers ask if I have a secret stash of happy pills hidden under the dark chocolate bars I hide in the kitchen pantry. The answer is no—unless, of course, you count Prêt à Manger's Honey Banana Granola Prêt pot of yogurt as a form of "pill." Instead, I live, breathe, and spread happiness, except when my parents call me ten times while I am in a meeting to ask me what train I am on to see them in the 'burbs.

I once read a study in the *New York Times* that said people have a preset level of happiness. They're either happy or they're not. Life disasters happen—death, divorce, illness, rejection—but eventually we all go back to our set level of happiness. I'd like to say I was born happy—probably because I was freed from the sticky suffocating womb after nine entire months (it was really ten months), but you get the picture. My dad drinks for both of us, my sister cries for both of us, and I'm happy enough for all of us, for my whole family. Sometimes I wonder, am I so happy because I eat so much? After a lot of deliberation I've decided I'm happy partially because I was born happy and partially because I eat happy foods. If you weren't born with my genes, you can still be happy. That's where the food part comes in.

People, food is a privilege. In our family, it is our pride and joy. We don't feel guilty about it; instead, we enjoy it. Cooking together is an experience. It helps build a bond with our loved ones.

Believe it or not, food has the ability to do much more than pack a few pounds onto our bellies. Forget fad diets, forget sucky relationships, forget antidepressants, forget sex (well, maybe not forget), but really, forget all the crap you think "can make you happy," and realize the ingredients to happiness are staring you in the face the minute you enter your own kitchen.

In my kitchen, there are certain foods, five in particular, that give me an extra boost especially on my bad days—which I hardly seem to have now anyway simply because of what I consciously put in my mouth.

Numero uno on my list is oily fish. Trust me; I would never suggest anything oily like deep-fried McDonald's fries for happiness. But in this case, the fish works. I prefer salmon for my oily fish. I eat it raw or cooked; either way the salmon remains rich in omega-3 fatty acids, which is proven by many studies to help lift the human mood. I must admit I refused to eat the scaly sea creatures until I was about twenty-one years old and went on my first blind date (pause for rolling of eyes). Well, my Rico Suave date was not so blind when it came to ordering for both him and me. He selected the mahi-mahi, which I immediately resented (a dead-dolphin dish?). But surprisingly, I loved it, and I've been eating fish ever since—who knew something good could actually come out of a blind date, eh?

Numero dos is beets. Beets for some reason make me oober goober happy. I have them in my salads and slow roasted at home with a few spices. The red beet is unique for its high levels of anticarcinogens, meaning it helps prevent all forms of cancer. Compared to other vegetables, beets are moderately high in carbs, but they are low in fat and an excellent source of folic acid (folic acid helps make red blood cells, is high in vitamin B, and helps execute much of our bodily functions). Beets are also loaded with antioxidants that help the body against heart disease and birth defects. Truth be told, a good beet always seems to give a steady rhythm to my day—pun intended.

From Chapter 5, Eating Muffins Gives You Muffin Top, you already know that I lived off of cereal as a child; therefore I became very fond of milk. Soon this fondness matured, and turned into yogurt, making it numero trés on my happy list. If you've ever had a gyro or gone out for some pitas and falafels, you know one form of Greek yogurt already: tzatziki. Tztaziki, Greek yogurt paired with garlic, spearmint, and lemon, is used to top most meats in Greek cuisine. You can even add cucumbers to it—you'll never want to use sour cream or chunky blue cheese again (wide hips celebrate this wise decision to make you slim). But even as a snack, not only is Greek yogurt thicker and creamier than the disturbing moldy, liquid, runny texture of regular yogurt. Although it is not lower in fat (unless nonfat Greek yogurt is specified on the container), it is more filling than standard yogurt due to higher protein content. I usually pair Greek yogurt with honey and nuts, or add it in the blender when making smoothies. Either way, it satisfies me and lightens my mood every time. Some say it's becoming my fetish . . . my food fetish, of course.

Numero cuatro is nuts—my power food. Some prefer the taste of them in bed (ha!), but nuts such as almonds, pistachios, cashews, and peanuts definitely satisfy my snack cravings. I keep them in my purse or stashed in the office. I guess you could say for as much chocolate I have at work, I also have lots of nuts. Fortunately my nuts never actually make me go nuts. Instead, they serve as "brain food" because they have a high content of omega-3 fats, which help improve the blood flow in our brain—clearly my nuts got me through Harvard Business School. They could be routinely found in my purse in a Ziploc bag, among a plethora of other Ziploc bags containing borrowed jewelry, my Invis-Align retainers, and Matchbox cars I bribe my nephew with so he'll agree to poop in the pot. Emerald also makes a 100-calorie cocoa-roasted almond pack that is perfect for train nibbling.

And last, but not least, numero cinco is dark chocolate. When I was a kid, my mom used write a note for me to take with me to birthday parties: "My daughter is allergic to chocolate. She will try to eat it but PLEASE don't let her." After many torturous years of trying to eat chocolate and ending up with hives and an upset stomach due to being allergic to cacao (the main ingredient in chocolate), my system surrendered. Yes, at the ripe old age of thirty I started eating chocolate and managed to hold it! There is a God. Now I can experience what others love so much. Chocolate truly does make humans happy. It contains anadamine, a brain chemical that brightens our mood. Although too much sugar is never good, the sugar in chocolate boosts our happy hormones, our endorphins. It's a good thing I overcame my misfortune and joined the rest of the chocolate-eating population.

So there it is. My mood is related to food. Because of my five special foods, I can keep calm even during calamity. I may talk a mile a minute, especially about food, but I am a genuinely joyful person and an optimist. My happy foods keep me this way. I never dwell on things and always find the positive in ultradepressed scenarios—from my friend losing her mom during 9/11, to my grandmother's battle with lung cancer, to my own relationship disasters. I always have hope and a positive outlook. With that hope, I cook. And at the end of my cooking, there is food, and in the food, there is happiness. Sorry to sound like the preacher's wife, but on a serious note, this is my truth. My drug is my food . . . it gets me high on life without any of that cannabis plant crap.

Depressed I am not. A crier I am not—save that for my sister. But an eater I am, and will always be.

Chapter 22

Breakup Binge

Staying Amazing When My Heart Is Breaking

The doorbell rang at 2:00 A.M. It was a high school night and I wasn't exactly the teen the local cops chased around town, so my parents didn't stir to answer it. I peered outside the door and there was my older sister, sobbing uncontrollably, wanting me to let her in. She had traveled all the way from the University of Pennsylvania and not just to see my pretty face. Actually, this was high school—I take that back—my not so pretty face. You could say I looked more like a feathered Farrah Fawcett haircut gone wrong with teenage acne. You get the picture. Anyway, it turns out she broke up with her boyfriend. He was cheating on her, with an attractive blonde, no less—go figure. This, of course, warranted much more than Kleenex tissue boxes. Instead, a midnight snack of dinner leftovers would be the perfect remedy.

For the next few days, my sister inhaled cookies, wolfed down potato chips, and had my mom heading to the supermarket twice in one weekend. She was breaking records; clearly aiming for the freshman fifty, not the average fifteen. By day two, I'd seen enough bloodshot eyes, running-nose gook, and contaminated tissues to last a lifetime. Still, nothing I said or cooked would stop her from stuffing her face.

I was traumatized by this experience and shaken up by the utterly obese consequences. What's the point of ever dating if you have to gain so many pounds for each breakup? Talk about tough love. Well, more tough for the scale, I suppose. Still, it wasn't until my first real love in my twenties that I got firsthand experience with what the demon called the "breakup binge."

I've always had a tough outer shell. It takes time and energy for me to open up in a relationship and share myself. Once in my life, on a completely blind date, I let my guard down, threw out my long wish list (e.g. height—above 6 feet 1 inch, i.e., above sea level in my book; education—minimum of one Ivy League degree, etc.), and acted on impulse as I discovered true chemistry with a stranger.

We looked like the model couple. Ya know the whole nine yards: a lovely house, a lovely car, and a lovely attempt at happiness. Friends chomped at the bit to get invitations to our five-course dinners. Our hair was perpetually windblown from our rides in our silver Mercedes convertible. Fancy parties and fancy vacations were a part of our daily life together.

But that was just the surface; deep down there was trouble in paradise. We fought like cats and dogs, only the bickering went far beyond dinner battles. We stooped to the lowest levels possible, personally attacking each other on an inhumane level. Our insults and nasty e-mail exchanges were never-ending. I learned that there are two types of men in this world. Type one, who makes you feel like you are the only woman in the room and type two, who notices every woman in the room but you. Mr. Greenwich was type two.

Our first real breakup was World War II reincarnated. Only this time the hotel room exploded instead of Pearl Harbor. And by exploded, I don't mean orgasmic. It was during a vacation to Monte Carlo for Prince Albert's Bal de L'été—more like a vacation to Monte hell, if you ask me. Many witnesses attest that we made quite a spectacle of ourselves. The night of the actual event I cried myself silly for hours till I managed to put on my clothes and show up at the black tie dinner. Seated at a table with my friends, just one table away from him, I simply stared at my plate. It was the first night of my life where food became inedible, pitiful, I know. I pushed the entrée around my plate like each part was some miniature skater gliding around the rink. Aromas that used to entice me gave me the urge to vomit, and in two weeks I pretty much dropped all the relationship weight I'd gained in the six months prior where he had insisted on dining out every night of the week. I felt like crap inside while my body lost its shape and feminine curves to boot.

Just when I thought the war had subsided and the dust was going to settle, I started to miss him. I missed our companionship the most; Friday movie nights with fresh popcorn (made by me, of course), Saturday tennis games where he had me running around the court like a crazy racket-holding lunatic, and waffle making (his specialty) on Sundays.

To fill this void, I turned to my oldest and best friend: food. No amount of chocolate chip cookies could console me. Not even dunked in milk. Brownies only put a smile on my face for thirty seconds, and a tub of ice cream became a prebedtime ritual. Late-night infomercial watching was much more fun with my own bowl of popcorn. I was proud to say I discovered a new oral fixation in the bedroom: popcorn. It tasted much better anyway.

My clothes stopped fitting and left a line around my tummy from being too tight, but I didn't care. I had a broken heart. Apple crisp, macaroni and cheese, baked ziti, and pizza were working hard to fix it. My feelings numbed as my waist expanded. Sadly, this cycle continued (I'm truly embarrassed to say how many times) for over three and a half years. Carrie had Mr. Big and I had Mr. Greenwich. There was no rational explanation as to why we thought breakups and makeups would eventually settle down into a stable relationship. Word of advice: if it doesn't work once, it's doubtful it's meant to work again.

So, on Valentine's Day in Miami, I realized that despite how much I loved him, we'd never spend eternity together. He'd had a string of meaningless relationships before meeting me and he was destined to continue this pattern after me. Surrounded by hot Latinas clad in semibirthday suits, I was inspired to break the spell of my usual breakup routine. This time around, I did it all different.

I started by writing a diary. I also wrote him a very long letter, which I never sent him. It started off by reminding him of all the good times we had together, shoveling our car out of the snow so we could go have burritos and quesadillas in the middle of a storm (you'd think we'd opt for hot cocoa from Whole Foods), hugging so tightly that it hurt when each of our dads got sick, lighting the fire in the living room to stay at home and enjoy conversations on freezing winter days, and playing badminton in our backyard all summer long. Next, I addressed all of our issues: his constant need to flirt with every girl in a fifty-mile radius, his insane habit of not letting me sit on our bed in my "street clothes" (me, a hustler? please . . .), the fact that he took longer to get ready than I did and that I had to have "house slippers" for the house and "outside slippers" for when I dropped the garbage by the driveway. DO NOT get me started on why I was taking out the trash instead of him! The letter went from romantic to reminiscing to outlining all the reasons why he was a complete douche bag and boy, did it feel good. Writing it down freed me from the negative energy and allowed me to feel drained of the bad emotions. I was once again happy to face each day with a smile. I cleared the air and my conscience by typing out the thoughts in my mind.

While he preferred champagne and casual sex to mending his insecurities after every breakup, I was determined to be my fabulous self, only better. I hit the gym, hard, but not too hard. We all know giving your treadmill a sweat bath is not very ladylike. While Bravo and breakups are a match made in heaven, I limited my reality TV intake and got my ass off the couch. Soon enough, the icky feelings started to dissipate and bad vibes turned into good vibrations. Read into that one if you like.

I kept reminding myself of the naked truth: I had bent over backwards to make Mr. Greenwich happy for years and he continuously repaid me by bending the next one over every time we broke up. He followed the philosophy that it takes getting under one to get over one. I just didn't need it anymore. There were the evil e-mails, threats to throw my stuff out of the window, and many more unpleasantries, but I didn't let it faze me. I was sure I would get through it all, only this time I'd have a booty that he would only dream of bouncing quarters off of.

I didn't look for solace in the baked goods aisle; instead, I cleared my cupboards of every bad food. I ate several light small meals a day and drank more water than a camel. Most important, during this emotionally volatile time, I ceased my friendship with red wine and decided I would revisit my nights with her once I was feeling completely mentally sane. I threw myself into work, full force, and became busier than my busiest self (if you don't know me, picture the energizer bunny on crack, no joke). I surrounded myself with friends and my friend Stacy suffered through IMing me at least ten times a day so I wouldn't feel the void of my previously daily chats with Mr. Greenwich.

I'm also happy to say that I didn't look for the next Romeo to take my mind off of my failed relationship. Instead, I spent time getting healthy from the inside out; mind, body, and soul. I truly believe that you can't be good in a relationship until you are 100 percent A-okay with yourself. You need to be complete on your own to actually be able to complete another person. So I went back in my closet to try on my outer shell for size. I also ignored my friends' suggestions to visit the world of e-Harmony and Match.com. Instead, I kept myself busy without relying on a man to occupy my hours. I was eating antioxidants, exercising like a gym whore, and my skin was glowing. Eat your heart out, Mr. Greenwich. This time around I didn't need to chase my breakup with bourbon. Nothing said "I'm over you" like looking better than I did the day I met you. Still, the next fish in the sea better come along with an invite to a top-notch steakhouse for dinner. I may have lost some pounds, but I definitely haven't lost my taste.

Chapter 23

Food Cures All

When Life's a Bitch, Grieve, Don't Gorge

My grandmother always used to say, some people have "haath me jadu," which translates to "magic in their hand." She told me that people are born with an innate sense of flavors and textures and can master cooking effortlessly. She had ten grandchildren, but she always told me I inherited her magic hand for cooking. Her food was divine and meals at her home were the glue that held our big family together. Although she never ate meat, she cooked it for all of us to enjoy. To her, everything was better with butter. I took notes on her elaborate recipes, hoping to share them with my own grandchildren one day.

After my grandfather suffered many strokes and finally passed away, she came to live with us for a while. I had always enjoyed seeing her for a few weeks at a time during the holidays or for two months during the summer, but it wasn't till she lived with us that I truly got to appreciate the warmth of her heart and the magic of her culinary creations. In the first few weeks of her stay, my parents picked up on her hacking dry cough, which grew worse with each day. Upon running some tests, we discovered that my grandma, who had never smoked a cigarette in her life, had lung cancer. In just a matter of months, her ailing frame grew weaker and her time usually spent in the kitchen became time spent in a hospital bed. I made a point of coming home from college as frequently as I could on the weekends and just spending quality time with her. She told me the most touching stories about her childhood and although she was suffering with intense pain, you'd never know it from her kind disposition.

Upon enduring as much treatment as she could, she returned to her own home and passed a few months later. I remember feeling like I had been punched in the stomach by a 1,000-pound bowling ball when my mom broke the news over the phone. I lost my appetite entirely. I lived at the Alpha Chi Omega sorority house, where our kitchen table was covered with every type of cookie and mounds of cereal, and our house mom cooked two gluttonous meals a day. In my depressed state, nothing looked nibble-worthy. In fact, the day my grandmother died, I gave up eating meat to honor her. Somehow, I just lost the taste for it—shocking, I know.

My grandmother's death was my first strongly emotional experience with death. Once I regained my appetite, food became an easy way for me to distract myself from my sadness. I grabbed on to sugary sweets and breads, which had me feeling as high as a caffeine-infused kite and as low as Bernie Madoff's current bank account. I looked to food for comfort. Like most other vegetarians, I was only left with sugary or carb-filled meal options at our sorority house or the deep-fried foods within my college dining halls. I took matters into my own hands and started making dinner for myself every night. My cooking fueled my popularity among my friends on campus, and I was truly lucky for this. Those girls let me vent and share all my feelings with them, supporting me as I mourned through the death of my grandmother. Today, they are still my closest friends. Only their therapy sessions have switched gears to boys and business. The rate per session has also upped from cheap wine and home-baked cookies to merlot and Dover sole. They became savvy food and wine connoisseurs while my cooking got better.

However, eight years after I committed to vegetarianism, a mind-boggling final exam at Harvard Business School convinced me and my friends that burgers and beer were the only remedy for our law-abiding burnt-out brains. We went to Bartley's in Harvard Square for burgers. Presented with a cheeseburger and sweet potato fries, I fearlessly dug in. Three days later, my not-so-much vegetarian body was still puking and pooping. The cheeseburger wreaked havoc on my system, but I broke my body in for more meaty meals to come.

Speaking of meat, I always made it despite the fact that I didn't eat it for eight years. (I guess I missed dead cattle more than I thought.) Even though I was committed to eating tasty tofu, I would still cook juicy steaks for my friends and family. My dad always loved my lamb chops in rosemary and garlic. In fact, one would guess that he ate a little too many of them. After quitting smoking, he packed on more pounds than we thought were possible. A lover of good food, it showed on his body. It also became a strain on his heart. After heart failure, breathlessness, diabetes, and other issues, our family became accustomed to many trips to the hospital. This time around, I learned to cope with my grief. While waiting for test results, my family would eat out of boredom at the hospital cafeteria—salty vending machine vinegar chips, pizza overflowing with grease and cheese, Snickers bars, bitter coffee doused in sugar and whole milk, and of course, any roll or donut we could find at the nearest gift shop or café.

Yet I tried to escape. I would go for walks around the hospital and in the parking lot. I'd go food shopping and make everyone's favorites to comfort them. My sister thanked me for my cauliflower soup when she got home from a long day at our dad's hospital bedside. Her kids ate my steak with chimichurri sauce— thank you to Aaron Sanchez for teaching me how to make the perfect chimichurri; you're not only a Food Network star, but a chef whose recipes put smiles on my family's tired faces.

Some people paint all night, or run miles through their neighborhood to cope with hard times. Instead, I paint cakes with sweet colored icing and run circles around my kitchen. I slave over the stove and put my heart into every ingredient I use. Cooking became my therapy and also gave me control over what I put in my mouth. In the roughest times of sickness, I found that making simple yet flavorful food would lighten the mood in our home, lift our spirit, and of course, satisfy our stomachs. I took over the role of my grandmother; my meals now served as the glue that held my family together. I can feel her smiling down on me from a better place.

Then one day, as I was boiling eggs at 11:00 A.M. while checking e-mails on my Mac, my mom called. That Monday, my dad had had a tumor removed from his throat. I was in meetings with NBC regarding our holiday programming and had missed the surgery. She'd been dodging my calls for a few days, so I was eager to speak with her. She was hesitant to make plans with me for lunch the next day and I could tell immediately from her voice, something was wrong. After a little pleading, a small dose of harassment, I got it out of her. "I can't leave Dad at home this weekend. He has cancer," she told me. That was all it took for me to eat one boiled egg, put the other one in the fridge, and pack my bag to head to my parents' house.

An hour later, I arrived in the driveway and my mom gave me the kind of hug that you give your child when you send them off to college. Yet this time I was no longer eighteen years old, and the hug meant more than just a good-bye and try to keep your legs shut in college. It was a hug full of extra loving and filled with pain all at the same time. We wiped the tears in our eyes and headed upstairs. My dad was sitting, as per usual at his desk, just staring at his computer. I asked him, "Dad, how are you feeling?" He replied, "I'm okay. It is what it is." I broke down in uncontrollable sobs as did my mother. He said, "Sit down," so I did, unable to resist the box of Kleenex calling my name.

"Let's have lunch," he requested.

"What do you feel like eating?" I asked.

"I want to have chicken with roasted chestnuts. I think Emeril Lagasse makes a good one. Do you think you can make that?"

"Sure, I can," I replied. I suddenly had a decent appetite and a bit more emotional stability.

I headed down the stairs toward the kitchen smiling with a bit of relief. Once again, I knew I'd be cooking my way through cancer.

Chapter 24

Mr. Martini

Through the Kitchen Is
the Only Way to My Heart

My mother, who is determined to not let me die in spinsterdom, uses her incredible IQ when it comes to three things: snacking, gardening, and setting me up on the worst dates known to mankind, or should I say womankind? I believe her formula is to walk down a random street and pick the most hideous, hit-by-a-bus looking pseudo-intellectual and tell him about her daughter who works in Manhattan. I think she secretly wishes she was Cupid, and uses Manhattan as her love arrow. Well, the Cupid act is an epic fail, always. From the looks of these guys, you'd think she's exacting a horrible payback for a mischievous childhood sin—a bite of chocolate or a bowl of sugary cereal.

My sister, on the other hand, fares only slightly better under the Cupid mask. Her strategy involves quantity instead of quality (thank God she doesn't work in retail anymore). She simply asks every other school mom or social acquaintance if she has a single brother or cousin, as if it makes for wonderful coffee conversation every time. She's hit about every resident in her neighborhood, so she has moved on to in-boxing every Facebook friend now.

While I give my sister an A for effort, she deserves a D for results. I often remind her that at work, I pay people for results, not effort (I'm a business women, not a first grade teacher). In an attempt to redeem herself from her near failing grade, she finds it necessary to ask every partygoer at an event if they have a "single friend for her single sister." Mortified I am not. I am simply used to this behavior bordering on lunacy. By now I'm convinced it's genetic.

I left the party at 2 A.M. without meeting Prince Charming but I received a mysterious e-mail four days later that read, "We should grab a drink sometime." I replied, "Who is this?" To which he wrote, "Your sister gave me your e-mail. She is friends with my sister and I guess we missed each other at the party over the weekend." Embarrassed by my e-mail, I felt obligated to go for a drink. Obviously NOT TOO obligated because I set it up for a Monday night, wore leggings and a long sweater accompanied by unwashed hair, and not a stitch of makeup. If it were an eighties workout theme party, I'd be set. All too ac-customed to my sister's set ups, I decided that ten minutes of inserting contacts and wearing makeup would be a poor use of time. Instead, I zipped through ten more e-mails at my desk and went on my way.

Mr. Martini sucked down two dirty ones in the time I sipped three-quarters of a glass of Pinot Noir. He was surprisingly handsome (props to my sis) and very fun loving. Despite the fact that the conversation was flowing (just like his drinks), my stomach was letting out old-lady growls: the really loud kind when you haven't eaten for four hours and you have too look around to pretend to question where the animal noise is coming from. Convinced that things were going like any normal first date, I was gearing up for my free dinner, which is normal date protocol after the first cheap-ass drink date. I, however, turned out to be entirely wrong. Mr. Martini was satisfied with his buzz and didn't bother to offer to take me out for a bite. He left me standing alone like the kid who gets picked last for dodgeball. Only this time I was left on the streets of New York rather than on a playground where I could go on the swings and grab an ice cream cone to make me feel better (God, I miss being young).

His poor form allowed his ranking to drop precipitously (strike 1) until I got an e-mail from him the next afternoon: "Let's have dinner." Then I realized, he wasn't a jerk, he was just slow. Alcohol kills brain cells, ya know. Dinner the following week was my pick and his American Express treat. We bonded over rustic Greek bites including htapothi scharas (grilled, marinated octopus) and psari sta karvouna (classic grilled whole fresh fish). His irresistible charm and wit put me at ease. While I had put fifteen whole minutes into assembling my outfit and shaping my wavy hair into organized, not turbulent waves, Mr. Martini put me to shame with his dapper style.

On date number five he professed that women often asked him about what not to do in relationships. If I could have scratched my head at the table, I would have, but I have good table manners. I did some inner head scratching, though, and thought: He is a guy's guy, a true bachelor, a man in need of reform. Why would women ask a forty-year-old bordering on metro sexual single man for relationship advice? Regardless, a business lightbulb went off in my head at this very moment. I was practically beaming as I realized how valuable the crowds' wisdom on all things NOT to do would be in saving time and face in sticky situations. Mr. Martini probably assumed from my glowing face that I had a little too much to drink, or that I was head over heels for him. In reality, I was drunk off of yet another new dream. Head over heels for my second business. In that moment www.whatnottodo101.com was born.

Feeding me with a business idea was not Mr. Martini's only good deed. He took great care of me, made me laugh on an hourly basis, and tolerated my unforgivable work schedule, as he had one that was equally unbearable (workaholics attract I guess). More than anything, he gave me a reason to come home after a 12 to 15 hour work day and start cooking. Unfortunately, his kitchen was in the original condition it had been when his apartment building was built circa 1960. It took me two months to get him to confess that he did not know how to use the dishwasher, at which point I had to lay down the law. He had to remodel his Formica palace and replace it with a stainless-steel modern heaven if I was going to lift a finger in the kitchen. I was given the task of choosing the tile and cabinet design, which was of course, a plus.

My wish was granted (as were many more) and meals started to flow. As long as the chicken didn't have bones, there was no basil in sight, and cheese was omitted for him to maintain his cholesterol, he would smile (you know it's serious if I accept the ridiculous no basil and cheese diet).

Preparing dinner on weeknights and lunch on weekends for him was easy, which left me more time for dessert.

By now I've learned that food is the key to every relationship, whether it be with a man, my family, my friends, or myself. Cooking releases me and gives me happiness I can't get anywhere else. At your next meal, stop calculating in your head the hundreds of calories on your plate. Instead, feel energized by the good choices you've made and savor a few bites of the decadence you deserve. Cherish the reasons you love sharing the yummy bites in front of you with the person seated across the table. Remember that food can bring people together at the biggest celebrations and in the most difficult times. You will laugh, joke, cry, reunite, or even fall in love over many meals in your lifetime, so food will always be good company to keep. And as for Mr. Martini, I may or may not need a man, but I will always need a good kitchen.

Acknowledgments

My life is my business. My business is my life. They are one and the same. Since the day I thought of the idea for Behind the Burner, not a single day has passed by without working. It might sound boring to you but it has been the most exhilarating and exciting experience of my life. So, naturally, when I thought about writing a book, I wrote a proposal for a Behind the Burner book filled with tips, tricks, and techniques for food. My agent, Kate Lee, whose cooking involves not cooking at all (carrots and hummus counts as a meal at home), tried to prevent her eyes from rolling back into her head. Kate and I became fast friends and she took me straight to Julia Cheiffetz and Katie Salisbury at HarperCollins. Julia and Katie, like Kate, believed in me, my vision for the company, and all the exciting opportunities I had in the works. Although they didn't *love* my idea for the book, they took a bet and reeled me in. At our first editorial meeting, after I had poured hours of carpal-tunnel-inducing typing into my manuscript, Julia suggested I try to write a few sample chapters for an entirely different book: one about me. Both scared and inspired by the challenge, I wrote the samples. Julia, Katie, and Kate all liked them; hence, *Sexy Women Eat* was born. Thank you for taking some risks, and most of all for having faith in me.

I wrote the first draft of this book at the one place where I could get the most inspiration: my parents' kitchen table. With easy access to the stove and fridge, I prepared lots of tasty nibbles that let my creative juices flow. Thank you, Mom, for convincing me to take short breaks and go for walks with you. I needed the exercise but always enjoy your company. Also, thanks for only complaining about how much I work 85 percent of the time. One day, I hope you will realize that my drive and ambition are here to stay and they truly make me who I am. Still, you are largely responsible for shaping my morals, beliefs, and ethics and for that I am incredibly grateful. You may not know this, but I actually read your five-paragraph-long spiritual e-mails, filled with typos (apparently, they run in the family), encouraging me to be a better person, live without worldly desires, and do good for humanity. You continue to send them to me, despite me telling you I automatically delete them, which tells me my insane persistence and perseverance must come from you. My father, unlike my mother, doesn't get calls from the local bank branch manager asking him why he signed his check with a calligraphy pen, so I must have inherited my common sense and street smarts from him.

Furthermore, this book would not have been possible if it wasn't for my *amazing* team, most notably Joanna Weinstein, Alix Weiner, Aditi Malhotra, Kaitlin Lipe, Lisa Curry, Jennifer Ambrose, Mona Buehler, Celeste Hughey, and Emily Rodney.

They are my heart and soul. My sister read each chapter in painstaking detail to refresh my memory on all of my awkward and humorous moments where she laughed at me, not with me—a common occurrence in our sisterhood. She is actually infinitely funnier than I am, and if she took a hot-second break from Internet shopping, she could probably write a book that would put mine to shame. Then again, she often reminds me that she does not "write," she "edits," and I should know the difference. Natalie Stein reminded me that I can't spell and marked up my manuscript in true lawyerly fashion. Many more friends (you know who you are), who would have volunteered to undergo multiple root canals before signing up to read drafts of my book, did me the favor of giving their input, suggestions, and advice that is peppered throughout the book. Better yet, Lisa Curry and Kaitlin Lipe tested all of my recipes, so if they don't work out for you, feel free to send them rotten tomatoes.

Please do judge this book by its cover. It was a labor of love and a lesson in analysis paralysis.

Thanks to Zanna Roberts (stylist extraordinaire), Karuna Chani and Stephanie Follari of KC Makeup, and Anna Shori (photographer), shooting the author photo was a piece of cake. Alba Cera, our food stylist, and Alix Weiner made sure I was never hungry, which was clearly the most important task of the day.

Finally, I can't tell you how thankful I am for the opportunity to tell my story. From buffets to board rooms, follow my advice. A positive relationship with food is a must. You can chalk up the inadvertent health benefits to sheer coincidence.

Just remember, *Sexy Women Eat*. They have an appetite for life.

Sources

Carb Counts for Avocados
Carbohydrate and Nutritional Information, by Laura Dolson,
   About.com Guide
www.healthdiaries.com/eatthis/10-health-benefits-of-apples.html
www.e2necc.com/egg-index.html
www.medicinenet.com/fiber/page3.htm#2CONTROLLING
www.campshane.com/nutritional/nutrition/fiber.htm
www.gutsense.org/reports/myth.html (myths to add to table)
www.crystalsugar.com/products/products5.sfacts.asp
www.avocado.org
www.cacaoweb.net/nutrition.html
http://emedicine.medscape.com/article/1182710-overview
www.marieclaire.com/health-fitness/weight-loss/shocking-
   eating-habits-statistics
www.healthcentral.com/diet-exercise/heart-diet-
   000043_2-145_5.html

About the Author

DIVYA GUGNANI is the founder and CEO of the culinary media brand Behind the Burner (www.behindtheburner.com) and What Not To Do 101 (www.whatnottodo101.com). She acquired a taste for her future in culinary arts while building a career in finance. In addition to a B.S. from Cornell University and an M.B.A. from Harvard Business School, Divya holds a degree from the French Culinary Institute, where she discovered her inner chef. She appears on NBC's *Weekend Today* and *New York Nonstop*, and MSNBC's *Your Business*. Divya contributes to The Huffington Post, The Daily Beast, Glo, and PageDaily. She has also been a guest on *Fox & Friends* and *TV Asia*, and has been featured in *BusinessWeek*, the *Wall Street Journal*, *The Deal*, *Crain's*, *Hi! Blitz*, *Khabar*, and *Time*, among several other publications. Follow her on Twitter (www.twitter.com/dgugnani or @sexywomeneat) or become a fan on Facebook of *Sexy Women Eat*.